Praise For:
Going Against Goliath

If there's one thing that Philip achieves in his book, it's giving hope! In dealing with cancer, hope is certainly not a luxury but a necessity. He also answers some very pertinent questions. Well done!

—**Leonard Stone,** Senior Pastor: *Maranatha Community Church*; National Leader of *The Christian Network (TCN)*, *South Africa.*

***

I enjoyed reading Philip's book—he has been my patient ever since he was diagnosed with Multiple Myeloma in 2017. I have witnessed first-hand his courageous battles against this disease which he refers to as his "Goliath." He shares valuable insights and medically sound advice out of the wealth of his personal experience. I believe that what he writes will be a source of encouragement and hope to any cancer sufferer.

—**Dr Sarita Retief,** Oncologist, Nelspruit Mediclinic.

***

In April 2018 Phil Robson and I were admitted to hospital to start our treatment for a rare and incurable blood cancer known as Multiple Myeloma. We didn't know each other at the time, and we certainly didn't know much about the challenges that lay ahead as we embarked on an intensive period of treatment involving a Stem Cell Transplant with high dose chemotherapy.

Since our discharge and through our recovery with various therapeutic treatments, Phil and I have bonded and we are in regular contact to assist each other as new challenges emerge. Phil has developed a superior level of knowledge about Multiple Myeloma, partly due to his previous encounters with cancer but also from his prior exposure to microbiology and genetics.

I was honoured to fact check Phil's book and found it reassuring that he was able to address the technicalities of cancer along with the spiritual, mental and practical challenges that patients face.

—**Gordon Russel,** Multiple Myeloma Patient, Former MD of *Haggie Rand, South Africa.* Retired business owner/manager.

***

Going against Goliath describes battles with cancer that demand physical, emotional and spiritual engagement.

As I read through this book my mind went to two specific things. Firstly, I remembered that in one of my last visits to Hatfield Church in Pretoria South Africa I shared on the story of David and Goliath and secondly that this story is personally relevant to our family. At the age of 16 our youngest son David contracted an aggressive cancer at the back of his right eye. Earlier in our church a prophecy was declared: "King cancer will be defeated." We entered severe battles that eventually resulted in his healing and deliverance. It was the most difficult time we have ever faced but we now have a testimony of God's faithfulness and healing power.

Philip's story, I am sure, will be a help and blessing to many. It's not an easy read but it carries wisdom and first-hand knowledge of how giants can be defeated.

—**Stuart Bell,** Senior Pastor of *Alive Church, Lincoln, UK.* Leader of the *Ground Level Network of churches.*

***

I have had the privilege of working closely with Phil Robson in our network of churches for many years and have witnessed his battle with three different types of cancer and his victories over the last number of years.

I found this book very interesting, informative and well balanced in the way that he married the spiritual with the natural in a unique way. I'm sure that everyone who reads it will find it very encouraging and useful.

When I was diagnosed with prostate cancer myself, Phil was very helpful in offering me sound advice, (much of which is found in this book), which helped me in the decision I made. Thankfully through much prayer and expert medical help I too have conquered my "Goliath."

I can fully recommend this book, especially to those still involved in their battle against cancer as well as to their loved ones.

—**Sid Hartley,** National Coordinator of *The Christian Network (TCN), South Africa.*

***

In *Going against Goliath* Phil Robson has provided the body of Christ with an inspiring, insightful and informative account of cancer surviving by means of his own encounter with this giant on three different occasions.

His practical and spiritual summaries at the end of each chapter are helpful and encouraging and will greatly aid both cancer sufferers and those who surround them in their journey.

Although each cancer journey is different due to the specific type and the individual, this book is highly recommended as a resource for the person who is personally *Going against Goliath*, their family and friends, and their pastors and counsellors.

—**Shaun Joynt,** Ph.D. in Practical Theology (Univ. Pret.) Facilitator: *Care Hub*, Pastoral Counsellor: *Hatfield Christian Church*.

***

Pastor Phil is well known in the small community of Sabie and many have rejoiced over his remarkable recovery from his various encounters with cancer.

As a cancer sufferer in remission myself, I'll admit I was a bit reticent to read Philip's book on battling cancer. I tended to want to push any thoughts on this matter as far from my mind as possible. However, reading the book inspired me to process my emotions further and to take courage. The reader will find much emotional, spiritual and practical help in these pages.

—**Letitia de Wet**, Manager and Senior Pharmacist, *Van Heerden Pharmacy, Sabie.*

***

In *Going Against Goliath* Pastor Phil does what good leaders do: he deals with reality and leads to hope. This book is a healthy description of how to holistically fight a battle with the giant of cancer. Pastor Phil writes about "faith facing facts," a real-world approach not only to the realities of our fallen, disease-affected world but also to the substantive hope Jesus Christ provides in our everyday lives. The interweaving of personal anecdotes, science, scripture, and faith make this book well worth a read.

—**Neil Bester**, Facilitator of Ministry Training and Organizational Development at *Hatfield Christian Church*.

GOING AGAINST GOLIATH

HOW TO FIGHT CANCER AND WIN!

Philip Robson

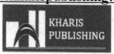

This book is dedicated to the many thousands who are facing and fighting the dread disease called Cancer. May my experience in engaging this enemy help you in your battle. May you move from being a victim to being a victor.

To my father: Stanley Robson

And my sister-in-law: Sharon Boyd

(Who both succumbed to cancer)

TABLE OF CONTENTS

Prologue

Despite her unwavering faith and her amazing, quiet, fortitude, I could see that my sister-in-law Sharon was busy dying. My wife Desi had committed to stand in faith alongside her sister and to trust God for her healing. She kept vigil at Sharon's bedside during the last days of her struggle. The two of them made a formidable team as they prayed together and listened to recordings of Scriptures regarding healing. Although I was more focussed on the realities of the disease than they were, I wasn't about to say anything to discourage their bold faith. I tried to ignore what my eyes were telling me as I also laid hands on Sharon and prayed for her healing as many others had done before.

Sharon had attended a Word of Faith church and had graduated from their Bible College. When she was diagnosed with breast cancer, she firmly decided to forgo any medical treatment. She meticulously followed a diet of healthy foods reported to have anti-cancer properties and fervently believed that God would heal her.

Earlier on in her illness, she took a long trip to Durban with other members of her church to attend a healing campaign by an internationally renowned evangelist. During the event, the man of God had a word of knowledge that God was healing women with breast cancer. Sharon responded and even went up onto the platform for prayer. Believers laid hands on her; she fell down under the power of God, and lay motionless for some time. When she arose she believed she had been healed.

Sadly, the disease progressed relentlessly, and Sharon wasted away before our eyes as her body became riddled with cancer. She died peacefully in her parents' home at age fifty. We were all devastated. My children adored their aunt, and Desi and Sharon had been very close. Participating in her memorial service proved to be a heart-rending experience for my family. Following this, Desi went through what one could call a "crisis of faith", and it took her some time to process her emotions and her disappointment at the death of her sister. The sad thing about all this was that the cancer had been diagnosed early on and the disease could have been treated successfully medically.

My story is somewhat different. I am a veteran cancer survivor. Over the past twenty years I have had to face and fight three different cancers: malignant melanoma, prostate cancer and more recently, multiple myeloma. I rejoice to report that malignant melanoma and prostate cancer are things of the past and that I have been in complete remission from multiple myeloma for some time. Like Sharon, I believe in divine healing and, as a pastor, I have witnessed some amazing miracles of healing through prayer during my thirty-five years of ministry. However, unlike Sharon I did not forego medical treatment. In this book I will explain why I see no conflict between exercising faith in a healing God and receiving the best modern medicine can offer. I will argue in favour of a holistic, multi-pronged approach to overcoming cancer which includes faith, prayer, medical treatment, the support of loved ones, diet and exercise.

I passionately hate this group of diseases collectively called 'Cancer' or also referred to as "The Big C," and want to encourage and provide practical help to all who find themselves facing and fighting this enemy. May you cut "The Big C" down to size!

Prologue

This book is also intended for friends, family, caregivers, as well as those in a pastoral or counselling ministries, supporting those with cancer. What I write will be of particular help to those who have been diagnosed with the same cancers that I fought, but the principles I unpack can be applied to any cancer.

On the one hand I have tried to provide a scientific explanation of cancer. Since I hold a science degree in microbiology and genetics and had several years of experience in a research environment before being called into Christian ministry, I am fortunate to be able to understand much of the scientific and medical jargon that is found in the literature about cancer. However, this is definitely not a textbook on cancer. My purpose is to equip you, the reader, with an understanding of the disease without being too technical. I will try to explain things as plainly as possible. In the interest of simplicity, I have purposefully stuck to citing cancer websites which explain things in everyday language. I have also summarised some of the key facts covered at the end of the more technical chapters.

On the other hand, I have tried to include my own spiritual experience with the disease. I have gained many spiritual insights through my years of ministry and my personal battles with cancer, and have arrived at what I believe is a balanced approach to healing and health. I am unapologetically Christian and believe that faith in God plays a central role in overcoming cancer. Therefore, much of what I share will be inspirational in nature. I will share very openly about many of the personal challenges I faced and how I received comfort and encouragement through my relationship with God, and reading and believing the scriptures. I also summarise some of the lessons I learnt at the end of some chapters and include some example prayers to pray.

Although I write from a Christian perspective, I believe that what I share will help those of other faiths and may even inspire those who have not yet come to faith, not to fight their battles alone.

As you read these pages, may you be empowered and inspired to "Go against Goliath." It is my prayer that this book will help you learn how to fight cancer - and win!

CHAPTER 1

ENCOUNTER WITH A CROW

I t had been an amazing time in the presence of God with a bunch of enthusiastic young believers. As a young Christian, eager to learn and full of zeal, I had booked into one of Youth with a Mission's (YWAM's) two-week discipleship training courses during my December college vacation. The teaching impacted on my life, and the times of worship were what I imagined it would be like in heaven – out of this world!

Now, as the camp neared its end, I decided to go on a three-day fast to seek the Lord's direction for the rest of my life. The YWAM base was in the countryside and it was hot and dry. In fact, we were in the middle of a drought. On the third day of my fast I walked some distance into the parched, blistering veld and knelt in the dirt in prayer.

As I wrestled in prayer, something strange happened. I was startled by a loud whooshing sound as a crow dive-bombed very closely over my head. I lifted my head and watched as it climbed effortlessly into the sky. Shrugging my shoulders at this strange occurrence, I re-engaged in prayer.

It wasn't a minute or two later when not only did I again hear the same sound, but I actually felt the wind as the crow passed even more closely over my head. This time I stood to my feet and shouted, "Voertsek!" (The South African version of 'Push Off!').

Not to be deterred by the interruptions, I again knelt in the dirt and proceeded in prayer. Minutes later the crow returned yet again. This time its claws actually grazed through my hair. Incensed, I jumped to my feet and, grabbing some stones, I shouted and pelted the bird as it flew into the distance. It never returned!

I pondered what had prompted this strange behaviour from the crow. Perhaps I looked broken and helpless as I knelt in the dirt in a dry and hostile area, and it had mistaken me for "dead meat." However, I sensed that there was perhaps some deeper spiritual significance to this strange occurrence. The Lord showed me that the crow was a harbinger of the trials and temptations that I was to face in future. Hadn't Jesus faced three temptations by the Devil as He fasted in the wilderness? I was also reminded that these temptations increased in scope and magnitude? (You can read the account in Matthew 4:1-11)

The first temptation to turn stones into bread was to satisfy Jesus' own personal appetite for food. The second was to jump from the pinnacle of the temple to prove the Father's angelic protection and to win the adulation of the religious crowd. The third temptation promised Jesus that He would own all the kingdoms of the world. It is significant that Jesus rebuffed each of Satan's temptations by saying, "It is written…" and then quoting a relevant Scripture from the Word of God.

I carried a lasting lesson away from this encounter: it seems that temptation often arrives when one is most vulnerable and that often it consists of a season or series of temptations. Jesus was tempted by the Devil for a full forty days, and the three temptations listed arrived at the culmination of this contest. Luke's account ends with the words:

> **When the devil had finished all this tempting, he left him until an opportune time.** —Luke 4:13

Many years later when I faced my third and most serious cancer diagnosis, the Holy Spirit would remind me of this incident. Cancer, or "The Big C" as it is often called, is something dark and sinister that seems to descend on the unsuspecting out of nowhere just like the crow did.

In this book I will relate some details of my personal battles with cancer and hopefully equip you, the reader, to be more effective in your fight, should you be facing the same enemy.

CHAPTER 2

WINDS OF WAR

I was what one would call a "water baby." From a young age I loved swimming and soon became very proficient at it. From merely playing in the water, I soon graduated to serious swimming and spent countless hours training under various coaches during my school years. I swam in numerous galas and was fortunate to win many events and even held some records in my junior and high schools, and then in the greater city of Germiston where I grew up.

In those days we didn't have the very effective water-proof sunscreens available today, and being of English stock, I was fair skinned and often ended up sunburnt. I was what the Afrikaners called "'n regte rooinek" (lit. a real red neck, a somewhat derogatory term for the English)

In later years, my skin started to pay for my negligence of it, developing cancerous lesions which led to periodic visits to a dermatologist. He would then enthusiastically "burn off" any lesions and sores on my skin with liquid nitrogen and I ended up looking rather battle-scarred. I would joke afterwards that I had had a fight with my skin specialist and that he had won!

On a couple of occasions, he dealt with more serious cancerous lesions. He removed both a Basal Cell Carcinoma and a Squamous Cell Carcinoma. Both of these cancers are fairly slow moving and are not life-threatening if they are treated.

Malignant Melanoma

On one of my visits, I showed him a dark brown mole or melanoma which was developing on my left calf muscle. It was slightly raised and had grown noticeably in the previous few months. He didn't like the look of it and decided to remove it and send it in to a pathology laboratory for further investigation. He called me a few days later with the bad news that it had proven to be a malignant melanoma and said that he had made an appointment with a surgeon to have all traces of it completely removed. The news came as a bit of a shock, but the full import of it only began to sink in later when I gained an understanding of exactly how dangerous malignant melanoma could be.

After administering a local anaesthetic, the surgeon removed a sizeable chunk of flesh around the site of the melanoma. Afterwards he had to stitch me up. It was all done and dusted in under a half an hour. However, as an added precaution, my skin specialist had also arranged for me to see an oncologist who explained some of the dangers of the disease once I visited him. He said he was confident that we had caught the melanoma at an early stage, but warned that there wasn't really any effective treatment against this sinister class of cancer.

Oncologists have few effective chemotherapy agents in their arsenal and radiotherapy is not an option. The only treatment that had shown a little promise at that time (2003), was a high dosage treatment of Interferon for a couple of years. When I say, "little promise," I mean it had only been shown to improve a patient's chances of survival by three percent. (Interferon is naturally produced by the body in our immune response to disease, but in this case it would be administered at something like a hundred times the dosage in which it would normally occur.) Understandably, my wife Desirée (I affectionately call her Desi) and I left the appointment rather fearful and discouraged.

On reading up about Malignant Melanoma, I discovered that it was regarded as the most dangerous of the skin cancers because it could spread very quickly and be lethal.

Melanoma is a serious form of skin cancer that begins in cells known as melanocytes. While it is less common than basal cell carcinoma (BCC) and squamous cell carcinoma (SCC), melanoma is far more dangerous because of its ability to spread to other organs more rapidly if it not treated at an early stage. (Skin Cancer Foundation. 2020)

Some call it the "ghost cancer" since, if given the chance, it can spread to and just appear in any part of the body, not just the skin. I began to realise that I had been visited by an intruding ghost. What evil exploits could I still expect from it? Because there are few effective treatment options, the disease often invokes fear in the patient. Interferon was also reputed to have horrible side-effects which would severely reduce the quality of one's life. It could prove worse than the disease itself.

According to Mayo Clinic (2020), there is a strong correlation between malignant melanoma and a high exposure to sunlight, but the ghost cancer follows no rules and people even experience malignant melanoma growths on the soles of their feet which rarely see the sun. Nevertheless, as a precaution against further melanomas developing, the oncologist advised that I use sunscreen liberally on every exposed part of my skin whenever I went outdoors.

God Speaks

As a follower of Christ and believer in the God of the Bible, my first recourse was to pray before making any decisions about treatment. A key verse from the book of Proverbs has been helping me to stay on course through the years, and proved very relevant under these circumstances:

> *Trust GOD from the bottom of your heart; don't try to figure out everything on your own. Listen for GOD's voice in everything you do, everywhere you go; he's the one who will keep you on track.*
> —Proverbs 3:5-6 MSG

Receiving guidance from God begins with trusting in the LORD– God is trustworthy and our faith pleases Him. It involves our hearts more than it does our minds. You have to choose to be led by your heart rather than by your head. Does this mean that we commit intellectual suicide and don't use our common sense? No, not at all! The book of Proverbs is also full of down-to-earth wisdom and common sense and it encourages us to take only paths that are firm. However, there needs to be a place for intuition as well as for reason; there needs to be a place for the word of the Lord over and above the opinions of men. Which one are you leaning on?

I remember kneeling on the carpet in the front of our beautiful church auditorium in a tumult of emotions with various questions crowding my mind. 'Why me, Lord? Have I not dedicated my life to serving You and Your people? Has something I've done displeased you?' As I poured out my heart to God, I began to experience His comfort, and peace started to settle on me. Then a voice spoke to me on the inside saying, *"Trust me for your healing, I can do a whole lot better than three percent!"*.

Through practice in listening to God over the years, I had learned to recognise this inner voice as what many refer to as 'the still small voice of the Holy Spirit.' God doesn't necessarily speak through the spectacular; He often speaks in a gentle whisper as was the case with Elijah when he fled from Queen Jezebel to Mount Horeb.

The LORD said, "Go out and stand on the moun-tain in the presence of the LORD, for the LORD is about to pass by." Then a great and powerful wind tore the mountains apart and shattered the rocks before the LORD, but the LORD was not in the wind. After the wind there was an earthquake, but the LORD was not in the earthquake. After the earthquake came a fire, but the LORD was not in the fire. And after the fire came a gentle whisper. When Elijah heard it, he pulled his cloak over his face and went out and stood at the mouth of the cave. Then a voice said to him, "What are you do-ing here, Elijah?" —1 Kings 19:11-13

I took action on the guidance I had received. At my fol-low-up appointment with the oncologist, I told him that I would be declining any treatment and that I would be trusting God for my healing. The meeting ended rather abruptly and acrimoniously with him asking why I had bothered to go and see him in the first place since I was unwilling to heed his advice. He seemed to feel that there was some direct conflict between exercising faith in a heal-ing God and receiving medication and that if one chose one option, one, by default, was rejecting the other.

You too might have to make the difficult choice be-tween treatment and simply exercising your faith. In mak-ing this decision it might be helpful to consider the follow-ing…

Faith versus Medicine

Am I anti-medication? Is there any conflict between exer-cising faith and taking medication? In answer to this ques-tion, I can state unequivocally that I see no such conflict. I only refused treatment in this instance because I believed I had a direct Word from God to do so. Also, the treatment suggested seemed very ineffective, would have negatively impacted on my quality of life and seemed to be an overkill given that we had caught the cancer at an early stage.

In answer to our question though, I am reminded of the healing of King Hezekiah which we read about in 2 Kings 20:

> *In those days Hezekiah became ill and was at the point of death. The prophet Isaiah son of Amoz went to him and said, "This is what the LORD says: Put your house in order, because you are going to die; you will not recover." Hezekiah turned his face to the wall and prayed to the LORD, "Remember, O LORD, how I have walked before you faithfully and with wholehearted devotion and have done what is good in your eyes." And Hezekiah wept bitterly. Before Isaiah had left the middle court, the word of the LORD came to him: "Go back and tell Hezekiah, the leader of my people, 'This is what the LORD, the God of your father David, says: I have heard your prayer and seen your tears; I will heal you. On the third day from now you will go up to the temple of the LORD. I will add fifteen years to your life. And I will deliver you and this city from the hand of the king of Assyria. I will defend this city for my sake and for the sake of my servant David.'" Then Isaiah said, "Prepare a poultice of figs." They did so and applied it to the boil, and he recovered.*
> —2 Kings 20:1-7

A few things stand out for me as I read this portion of Scripture. First, the news from the prophet Isaiah was really bad, *"This is what the LORD says: Put your house in order, because you are going to die; you will not recover." (v1)* This sounds like a death sentence to me!

(**Note:** When the oncologist looks across at you with a grave expression on his/her face and gives you the bad news, please realise that this is not the end of the story.)

Undaunted by this, Hezekiah prayed to the LORD and wept bitterly. If there is something that touches the heart of God, it is the cries and the tears of his children. (Let God know exactly what you are feeling; the psalmist David often did). In response, God seemingly changed His mind, and Isaiah was sent back to king Hezekiah with the message, *"...I have heard your prayer and seen your tears; I will heal you..." (v5)*

Then there was a practical step that was taken: Isaiah advised the application of a poultice of figs, a form of primitive medication. This probably drew out the boil which no doubt burst, releasing the infected pus resulting in Hezekiah's healing.

Jesus and Medicine

When we consider the healing ministry of Jesus it is evident that he too used what was considered effective medication in those days. In this way the Son of the Most High accommodated himself to the limited understanding of the sons of men. We read this report concerning the ministry of the twelve disciples whom Jesus sent out:

> **They went out and preached that people should repent. They drove out many demons and anointed many sick people with oil and healed them.**
> — Mark 6:12-13

Olive oil was symbolic of the Holy Spirit, but was also considered to have healing properties. Anointing the sick with oil and healing them apparently went hand in hand. Although no mention is made in the Gospels of Jesus personally administering oil, it is safe to assume that his disciples did so by following his example. In the story of the Good Samaritan, Jesus tells how the Samaritan took care of the man who fell into the hands of robbers:

> *But a Samaritan, as he travelled, came where the man was; and when he saw him, he took pity on him. He went to him and bandaged his wounds, pouring on oil and wine. Then he put the man on his own donkey, took him to an inn and took care of him.* —Luke 10:33-34

Oil and wine were considered to have healing properties and were medicines of the day.

Jesus also used his spittle in a number of healings; for instance, in the case of the man born blind.

> *...he [Jesus] spit on the ground, made some mud with the saliva, and put it on the man's eyes. "Go,"* he told him, *"wash in the Pool of Siloam" (this word means Sent). So the man went and washed, and came home seeing.* —John 9:6-7

The man's faith and obedience no doubt played a key role in his healing, but why the use of saliva? Could saliva have healing properties? This is not an isolated incident. On at least two other occasions Jesus used a similar methodology. *(See also Mark 7:33 and Mark 8:23)*.

In my opinion, saliva has definite healing qualities; that is why in nature many animals lick their wounds. I've found that a good way of getting rid of warts is to put saliva on them periodically and to leave it to dry. Jesus seemingly employed the commonly used "medicines" of the day; agents believed to have healing properties. He did not drive a wedge between faith and the use of medicinal agents and neither should we.

The late John Wimber was of a similar opinion:

Whether or not these treatments possessed scientific healing qualities is not the issue. Jesus associated with medical treatments; in fact, he seemed to sanction them. (1986:151)

Having answered this pressing question regarding faith and the use of medicine, you may now be asking me, "So what happened to your problem with Malignant Melanoma?"

The End of the Matter

As a precaution, I agreed to the prescribed quarterly blood tests that would be able to detect if melanoma was spreading in my body. Jesus sometimes told those whom he healed to present themselves to the priests in order to verify their healing, so I had no objection to any confirmation that would come via blood tests.

Here we have the example of Jesus instructions to a leper:

Jesus reached out his hand and touched the man. "I am willing," he said. "Be clean!" Immediately he was cured of his leprosy. Then Jesus said to him, "See that you don't tell anyone. But go, show yourself to the priest and offer the gift Moses commanded, as a testimony to them." —Matthew 8:3-4

In my blood tests they were looking for a marker called S100B which, if present, would indicate the presence of melanoma. Thankfully, the first year's quarterly blood tests were all negative. Following that, I continued having six-monthly tests for a couple of years. They all came back negative – Praise God!

My first bout of cancer did not prove to be that serious at all – it was rather like the crow's first visit when it just whizzed over my head. Yes, there was the initial scare, but God's personal promise to me and His constant presence gave me courage. For a while I had a puckered calf muscle where the surgeon had removed the growth, but in time that disappeared all-together. I had come through the first round in my fight against cancer unscathed!

My comfort in my suffering is this: Your promise preserves my life. —Psalm 119:50

Lessons Learned
- We should seek guidance from God before making any major decisions such as which treatment protocol to follow.

- God often speaks to us in a "gentle" or "small" voice on the inside rather than through spectacular outside events.

- There is no real conflict between faith and the use of medication.

- Both the prophet Isaiah and Jesus used what were regarded as the medicines of the day in healing the sick.

Key Facts
- Excessive exposure to sun in one's youth can lead to problems with skin cancer later in life.

- Those with fair skin should make use of the large variety of very effective sunscreens on the market today.

- Those who have problems with skin lesions should make regular visits to a dermatologist to have them treated.

- Malignant melanoma is the most dangerous form of skin cancer but can be treated effectively if caught early.

Notes

1. Skin Cancer Foundation. 2020. Melanoma Overview. Online article at URL: https://www.skincancer.org/skin-cancer-information/melanoma/ Accessed 2020-05-29

2. Mayo Clinic. 2020. Melanoma. Online article at URL:https://www.mayoclinic.org/diseases-conditions/melanoma/symptoms-causes/syc-20374884 Accessed 2020-05-29

3. Wimber J with Springer K 1986. *Power Healing*. London: Hodder and Stoughton. Page 151

CHAPTER 3

A MORE CHALLENGING CONTEST

Time slips through our fingers all too quickly. I had completed three years of Bible College at Hatfield Christian Church in Pretoria, then as a young family, we had arrived in the beautiful little town of Sabie to pioneer a fledgling church in the December of 1985. Over the years Living Waters Christian Church had been growing and flourishing under God's favour and blessing and many precious people were added to the family of God.

It had been a great privilege to bring up our three children in the wholesome community of this country village surrounded by mountains and forests, with its crystal-clear streams and beautiful waterfalls. But now the calendar on our wall read 2007 and our children had left the nest to study further and to pursue their individual futures in the big wide world. Just my wife and I were left to rattle around in our four-bedroomed double story log cabin which I had built.

It was time to take stock and accept, or even embrace, the passing of time. At 53 years of age, I was still young at heart, healthy and energetic, but at this time of life one has to become more aware of potential health problems.

A Particularly Male Problem

One of the diseases that men over fifty need to be particularly aware of is Prostate Cancer.

The prostate is a small gland which produces semen and which sits below the bladder. It surrounds the urethra through which urine is passed.

According to an article in the World Journal of Oncology:

> **Prostate cancer is the second most frequent cancer diagnosis made in men (next to lung cancer) and the fifth leading cause of death worldwide. 1,276,106 new cases of prostate cancer were reported worldwide in 2018... Prostate cancer incidence and mortality rates are strongly related to the age with the highest incidence being seen in elderly men (> 65 years of age).** (Rawla 2019 § 10(2):63-89)

The problem with prostate cancer is that it may be asymptomatic at first and its development is often slow and insidious. Other men, however, have very clear symptoms, but live in denial and stubbornly refuse to seek medical advice until it is too late. The tragedy of this is that prostate cancer is very treatable if caught early. However, the opposite is also true: if the cancer metastasises and spreads to the bones or other organs of the body, the treatment options narrow down and the prognosis of the disease is less favourable.

I began to notice that I had difficulty passing urine. I eventually consulted my family doctor who did a physical examination and some blood tests and then referred me to a urologist. When there are problems with the prostate like inflammation, infection or cancer it produces an antigen which can easily be detected in the blood. Physicians take note of the Prostate-Specific Antigen (PSA), reading in the blood, as it can be fairly useful in tracking the progress of the disease.

(For further information on PSA see [3] and/or [4])

A More Challenging Contest

At this stage my PSA reading was around 10 (ng/ml) which was not deemed excessively high, but the urologist said we would need to keep an eye on it. Since I had an enlarged prostate, he prescribed a drug known as an alpha-blocker. Alpha-blockers relax smooth muscles, largely in the bladder neck and prostate and therefore assist in the passing of urine.

The drug helped alleviate my symptoms, but, as directed, I continued to make regular visits to my family doctor and to have blood tests to monitor my PSA. With time my PSA crept up to 12.5 and my urologist felt it necessary to investigate further by ordering biopsies. I was booked into a day hospital where 15 tiny biopsies were taken from my prostate under anaesthetic. I experienced considerable pain after the procedure and blood was found in my urine. A few days later I was very disappointed to be told the bad news that I definitely had prostate cancer. (2 of the 15 biopsies were positive for cancer). The supposed good news was that we had caught the cancer at an early stage, and I had a Gleason score of 6 which was considered a low reading. (To understand your pathology report and the significance of your Gleason score see [4]).

Again, as with my previous diagnosis concerning malignant melanoma, the full weight of the prostate cancer diagnosis didn't hit me right away. I guess I was in a bit of shock or numbed denial. However, as I began to ask questions and to ask Google and surf the internet, the reality of it began to sink in. This could leave me incontinent or undermine my male sexuality and my sense of manhood. This could even kill me. How does one process something as serious as this?

My male friend, if you are reading this book, have been diagnosed with prostate cancer, and are wondering how you will survive the ordeal, please remember that you are not the first man to walk this road. We men tend to keep things to ourselves and as a result we face many challenges alone but it is really helpful to talk to people who have already faced the challenge and to get their perspective on the problem. Since I am a fairly public figure, a number of men have come to see me over the years, and it has been my privilege to reassure them and to share my insights with them. Most, if not all of them, felt it beneficial to have shared with me. This is also one of the reasons I am writing this book.

Decisions, Decisions

My urologist explained that various treatment options were available to me. In fact, there were so many that they were a bit confusing. There were the options of surgery, radiation therapy or of chemotherapy. One could also have hormone treatment to suppress testosterone and slow down the progression of the disease. A fairly new approach at the time (2009), was that of brachytherapy, a procedure where small radioactive seeds would be inserted into the prostate to effect internal radiation and control the cancer. Someone quipped jokingly that with this treatment you could end up "glowing in the dark".

Cancer.net (2019) offers the following good advice:

Take time to learn about your treatment options and be sure to ask questions if something is unclear. Talk with your doctor about the goals of each treatment, the likelihood that the treatment will work, what you can expect while receiving the treatment, and the possible urinary, bowel, sexual, and hormone-related side effects of treatment. Men should also discuss with their doctor how the treatment options may affect recurrence, survival, and quality of life. In addition, it is important to discuss your doctor's experience with treating prostate cancer. These types of talks are called "shared decision making."

A More Challenging Contest

As a former scientist I was familiar with doing literature surveys and so I also began to read extensively on the internet. I would also recommend this course of action. However, one needs to be careful that one reads reliable articles that are not out of date. Thankfully, many of them are written in layman's language and are relatively easy to understand. It is always best to be well-informed about the treatment options available and their various pros and cons. This also enables you to ask intelligent questions when in consultation with your physicians. Please note the following warning:

> *Prostate cancer treatments may seriously affect a person's quality of life. These treatments can cause side effects, such as erectile dysfunction, which is when someone is unable to get and maintain an erection, and incontinence, which is when a person cannot control their urine flow or bowel function.* (Cancer.net 2019)

Given the above statement, one can see that the choice of an appropriate treatment plan is an especially important decision. For me as a fairly young man who was physically fit, surgery seemed to be the best option as it held the promise of total eradication of the cancer with greater life expectancy. Both my urologist's advice and what I had read, confirmed this.

Led by The Spirit

From the time I first had blood tests indicating an elevated PSA level, my wife and I were praying for divine healing from any potential prostate cancer. I also shared with others close to me who laid hands on me and prayed for me. However, my blood PSA continued to climb and I felt it was time to heed sound medical advice. I have learned over the years that God, the heavenly healer often chooses to use earthly doctors and physicians as His agents of healing. After all, it is He who has given humankind its gifts of knowledge and understanding of the workings of the human body.

Now, as I deliberated over the important decision regarding the best treatment option, I prayed for guidance from God, trusting that the Holy Spirit would be leading me in any decisions I would make. There are numerous promises in the Word of God regarding divine guidance such as the following:

> *I will instruct you and teach you in the way you should go; I will counsel you and watch over you.* —Psalm 32:8

> *Whether you turn to the right or to the left, your ears will hear a voice behind you, saying, "This is the way; walk in it."* —Isaiah 30:21

During this time my wife and I attended a pastors' gathering in the city of Pretoria and happened to pass the Urology Hospital (an entire hospital devoted to this facet of medicine, with some of the top specialists in the field). On the spur of the moment I decided to stop there to ask about some investigative work they had done on ultrasound treatment for prostate cancer. I waited only a few minutes in a reception area when a very pleasant lady asked if she could help me. I enquired about ultrasound treatment and she said that had proved ineffective. However, she suggested that she take me upstairs to see the urologist with the best track record in the building regarding the treatment of prostate cancer.

When we arrived at his consulting rooms the waiting room was packed with people, but undauntedly my escort took me to the receptionist and boldly asked if they would squeeze me in to consult the doctor for a few minutes. The receptionist shrugged her shoulders saying that that was impossible and pointed to the crowded room. Not phased one bit, my escort asked, "Do you know who I am?" It turned out she was the matron of the hospital. The upshot of the story was that within a few minutes I was in the doctor's office asking him my most pressing questions about having a radical prostatectomy.

This doctor had studied under some of the leading urology surgeons in the USA and had returned to South Africa with what he considered to be a more effective surgical procedure for performing a radical prostatectomy. There would be less blood loss than in the method employed by most South African surgeons and the recovery time after the operation would be shorter. The chances of losing bladder control and erectile function would also be minimised. (Note: This surgeon is now an expert in computer aided robotic surgery and uses this technique as his method of choice).

I was convinced that this whole encounter was God ordained and had a real sense of peace after my discussion with this doctor. I called his rooms shortly afterwards to schedule the operation. We are encouraged in Scripture to allow the peace of God to rule, be the umpire, or to guide us in the decisions we make. I certainly had peace in this instance.

The peace that Christ gives is to guide you in the decisions you make; for it is to this peace that God has called you together in the one body. And be thankful. —Colossians 3:15 GNB

Into the Fire

The day of the operation arrived all too soon and was attended by a bit of pre-surgery apprehension on my part. Fortunately, believers have access to Jesus, the Prince of

Peace who encourages us to come to Him when we are weary or burdened. Knowing that we are perfectly loved is the remedy for fear. As I prayed, the peace of God filled my heart and I knew that everything would go just fine.

Here are some Scriptures on which I relied:

> *Come to me, all you who are weary and burdened, and I will give you rest. Take my yoke upon you and learn from me, for I am gentle and humble in heart, and you will find rest for your souls. For my yoke is easy and my burden is light."* —Matthew 11:28-30

> *There is no fear in love. But perfect love drives out fear, because fear has to do with punishment. The one who fears is not made perfect in love.* — 1 John 4:18

> *Do not be anxious about anything, but in every-thing, by prayer and petition, with thanksgiving, present your requests to God. And the peace of God, which transcends all understanding, will guard your hearts and your minds in Christ Jesus.* —Philippians 4:6-7

The operation went well and I was soon recuperating in the hospital ward. The friendly nurses were very attentive and encouraging. I remember waking up in the morning to the sound of their praying and singing in the hallway when they changed shift. When some found out that I was a pastor, they came to me just to chat or for some counsel or prayer. They expressed amazement at how positive and peaceful I was in contrast to some other men who apparently cried like babies after the operation. Only the Lord can bring us through the fiery furnace like He did with Shadrach, Meshach and Abednego, without even the smell of smoke upon us.

A More Challenging Contest

It's not the pain of the operation that is the problem for many men, but the fear of the word "cancer" and the fear of the potential loss of their masculine, sexual identity. Many struggle with self-pity, depression and a loss of drive and sense of purpose. I too, had to fight these demons in the days to come.

Once my histology report had arrived, my doctor told me the good news that "all my boundaries had been intact". This meant that the cancer had not spread to the nerves or veins in the prostate or to the seminal vesicle. It had also not penetrated the membranous capsule that surrounded the organ. During the operation they had not found it necessary to remove the lymph nodes in my groin. It was unlikely that I would have any further problems with prostate cancer since the cancer had been completely excised. It was indeed all good news – praise God! Within four days I was discharged and Desi drove us home to our beloved Sabie.

It wasn't all plain sailing though; I still had a catheter and a bag which I had to move around with me. My family doctor removed my stitches at the appropriate time and a while later removed the catheter. Almost from the outset I regained bladder control which was a great relief. (I have other male friends who struggled for some months to regain control after their operations). However, a few days later I developed an inflammation of the urethra and experienced extreme discomfort passing urine. We ended up having to drive all the way to Pretoria for an emergency consultation with my urologist. Fortunately, it wasn't long before I was happy and healthy again. As the saying goes, "all's well that ends well"!

My urologist had warned that a radical prostatectomy was a major operation similar to the hysterectomy a woman would have and that it would take something like six weeks before I would be able to return to my normal lifestyle. I used the recuperation time to relax in bed and to catch up on some reading. I was able to return to my pastoral duties in about five weeks. In answer to our prayers, my blood results were excellent with a PSA of zero for the next several years until I stopped having tests.

This second bout that I had to fight against the enemy cancer cut a little deeper and was a more significant confrontation requiring greater faith and endurance on my part. It was something like the second encounter that I had with the crow many years earlier: it came so close that I heard and felt its wind. However, Jesus was true to His promise and did not leave me nor forsake me. All praise be to His glorious name!

> ...*God has said, "Never will I leave you; never will I forsake you."* —Hebrews 13:5

Lessons Learnt

- Allow the peace of God to guide you in the decisions you make.

- Don't feel obliged to receive treatment from the first physician you consult with, but search for a person with a proven track record.

- Trust in God's perfect love for you. He will never leave you nor forsake you.

Key Facts

- Prostate cancer is very prevalent among men especially those over fifty.

- Because its onset is slow and insidious, many men ignore the symptoms at their own peril.

- Prostate cancer is very treatable if caught early.

- Men over fifty should consult their family doctors periodically for a physical examination as well as for blood tests to monitor their PSA.

- Various treatments are available for those diagnosed with prostate cancer. The pros and cons of each procedure should be weighed up prayerfully and carefully.

- Read up on the subject so that you can ask intelligent questions.

Notes

1. Rawla P 2019. Epidemiology of Prostate Cancer. *World Journal of Oncology*. 10(2):63-89. Online article at URL:https://www.ncbi.nlm.nih.gov/pmc/articles/PMC6497009/ Accessed 2020-06-04

2. Mayo Clinic 2020. PSA Test. Online article at URL: https://www.mayoclinic.org/tests-procedures/psa-test/about/pac-20384731 Accessed 2020-06-04

3. National Cancer Institute 2017. Prostate - Specific Antigen (PSA) Test. Online article at URL:https://www.cancer.gov/types/prostate/psa-fact-sheet Accessed 2020-06-04

4. Association of Directors of Anatomic and Surgical Pathology 2017. Understanding Your Pathology Report: Prostate Cancer. Online article at URL:https://www.cancer.org/treatment/understanding-your-diagnosis/tests/understanding-your-pathology-report/prostate-pathology/prostate-cancer-pathology.html Accessed 2020-06-05

5. Cancer.net 2019. Prostate Cancer: Types of Treatment. Online article at

URL:https://www.cancer.net/cancer-types/prostate-cancer/types-treatment Accessed 2020-06-06

Chapter 4

What is Cancer Anyway?

In Bible times, leprosy was one of the most dreaded diseases. If one had leprosy, it meant one would be banished from society so as not to infect others. One would become untouchable and would have to warn people of one's condition by crying out: 'Unclean! Unclean!' Fortunately, due to an increase in knowledge regarding the disease, modern medicine and antibiotics, leprosy has almost been eradicated.

A modern-day disease which evokes a similar dread in people's hearts is cancer, or "The Big C" as some call it. Often, when people are diagnosed with cancer, they see it almost as a death sentence. Knowledge is the key to understanding cancer and curbing the fear of the disease. It will therefore be appropriate for us to address a few questions about it before we proceed. The first thing we need to understand is what happens to the cells in our body when they become cancerous.

Each Cell Has a Function

Our bodies are fearfully and wonderfully knit together. David celebrates this in Psalm 139.

> *For you created my inmost being; you knit me together in my mother's womb. I praise you because I am fearfully and wonderfully made; your works are wonderful, I know that full well.* —Psalm 139:13-14

As a little baby forms in its mother's womb a process of differentiation takes place as cells take on various characteristics. Organs and structures develop as different genes in our chromosomes are switched on or off. A whole area of study in molecular genetics is dedicated to try and understand the control mechanisms that orchestrate this process. Scientists are only just beginning to understand how these processes work.

Although they all carry the same genetic code, the different cells in our bodies have totally different functions and totally different properties. For example, liver cells are responsible for cleansing and detoxifying the blood, whilst red blood cells are designed to carry oxygen to the tissues. Nerve cells convey tiny electromagnetic signals, whereas muscle cells are designed to contract at the impulse of nerve signals… and so we could go on. Each type of cell has a particular function and to fulfil this function a certain set of genes is switched on whilst another set of genes is switched off.

A cancerous or malignant growth begins to develop when the genetic code of a cell in a particular organ mutates or is damaged and as a result the cell loses its original identity and function. The cell's control mechanisms are somehow compromised and a "rogue cell" with no function or purpose results. In malignant tumours, such rogue cells begin to multiply and become a threat to normal, healthy cells. In aggressive cancers, the cells multiply very rapidly and may spread to various parts of the body very quickly.

Cancerous growths consume oxygen and nutrients and can even exert physical pressure within a given organ causing it to become dysfunctional.

Cancer kills by invading key organs (like the intestines, lungs, brain, liver, and kidneys) and interfer-

ing with body functions that are necessary to live.
(American Cancer Society 2020)

Healthy cells are an asset to the body since they fulfil a certain function, whilst cancerous cells are a huge liability since they compromise the health and even have the potential of destroying the life of the body.

An event in the life of Jesus illustrates what I am trying to say. It is the account of Jesus cursing the fig tree which bore no fruit.

> *The next day as they were leaving Bethany, Jesus was hungry. Seeing in the distance a fig tree in leaf, he went to find out if it had any fruit. When he reached it, he found nothing but leaves, because it was not the season for figs. Then he said to the tree, "May no one ever eat fruit from you again." And his disciples heard him say it.* —Mark 11:12-14

> *In the morning, (the following morning) as they went along, they saw the fig tree withered from the roots. Peter remembered and said to Jesus, "Rabbi, look! The fig tree you cursed has withered!" "Have faith in God," Jesus answered. "I tell you the truth, if anyone says to this mountain, 'Go, throw yourself into the sea,' and does not doubt in his heart but believes that what he says will happen, it will be done for him. Therefore, I tell you, whatever you ask for in prayer, believe that you have received it, and it will be yours.* —Mark 11:20-24

Cancerous growths in our bodies are like the branches of this fig tree which produced only leaves and bore no fruit. They deserve to be cursed since they have no function or purpose within the body. Jesus taught us that there is power in what we say; we can speak to the mountain of cancer and tell it to be removed. I believe one can and should literally curse cancer cells. I do so on a regular basis. I speak death on any cancer cell proliferating in my body and speak life over the healthy cells.

> **The tongue has the power of life and death, and those who love it will eat its fruit.** —Proverbs 18:21

> **Words kill, words give life; they're either poison or fruit—you choose.** —Proverbs 18:21 MSG

We have a traditional idea that prayer is asking for God to intervene, but in this instance the onus is on us to take a stand, speak to the mountain and curse the cancer cells.

How to Curse Cancer

(Focus on the Lord Jesus)

Lord Jesus, I know that all authority in heaven and on earth has been given to you, and I thank you that you have also delegated authority to me so that there is power in my words.

(Deliberately turn your focus on the disease)

Now, I address this disease called cancer in the name of Jesus and I command it to be cast out of my body. I curse any and every cancerous growth in my body and say that you will shrivel up and die. I speak death over every cancerous cell; you will not grow or multiply and I speak life over every healthy cell in the name of Jesus Christ the life-giver. Amen

What is Cancer Anyway?

Cancer is a Generic Term

As I have already said, one simple word that evokes much fear is the word 'cancer.' I guess it does so since cancer is the second-leading cause of death in the world. However, we should realise that the word cancer is a generic term for a whole range of diseases. Depending on which source you consult, you will discover that there are over a hundred different classes of cancer each with various sub-categories.

Cancer refers to any one of a large number of diseases characterized by the development of abnormal cells that divide uncontrollably and have the ability to infiltrate and destroy normal body tissue. Cancer often has the ability to spread throughout your body. (Mayo Clinic 2020)

Cancer is not one disease. It is a group of more than 100 different and distinctive diseases. Cancer can involve any tissue of the body and have many different forms in each body area. (Shiel 2018)

Cancer is often referred to simply by the name of the organ in which it occurs. So, in layman's terms we refer to lung cancer, brain cancer, liver cancer, pancreatic cancer, stomach cancer etc. The medical fraternity, of course, has many more complex descriptions for the various types of cancer which plague the human race. What we must remember when we hear the word cancer, is that not all cancers are equally dangerous to our health. Some are slow-growing and very treatable, whilst others are very aggressive and spread rapidly. (Just like there are harmless snakes and dangerous ones).

Earlier in this book I referred to my frequent visits to a dermatologist. Many forms of skin cancer are relatively harmless; no more than wart-like growths on our skin.

They tend to proliferate as we grow older. My skin specialist killed many of these by freezing them with liquid nitrogen. In the course of time he also surgically removed a Basal Cell Carcinoma and a Squamous Cell Carcinoma. Both are a bit more serious. They are not immediately life-threatening but need attention. Then came the more serious Malignant Melanoma or "Ghost Cancer", the subject matter of a previous chapter.

I urge you therefore, not to be seized by fear at the very mention of the word "cancer." Why should one word evoke such a knee-jerk response? Face whatever threat there may be with courage born of faith.

Over and over in the Word of God, we are encouraged not to fear. Here is a good example which has bearing on the healing of sickness and infirmity:

> *Tell fearful souls, "Courage! Take heart! GOD is here, right here, on his way to put things right and redress all wrongs. He's on his way! He'll save you!" Blind eyes will be opened, deaf ears unstopped, lame men and women will leap like deer, the voiceless break into song. Springs of water will burst out in the wilderness, streams flow in the desert.* —Isaiah 35:4-6 MSG

We need to take charge of our hearts to ensure that they are not given over to fear. *Above all else, guard your heart, for it is the wellspring of life.* **(Proverbs 4:23)**

Shortly before Jesus went to the cross which was followed by His return to heaven, He said these words to His disciples: *"Do not let your hearts be troubled. Trust in God; trust also in me...."* **(John 14:1)**

A heart left to itself will be prone to being troubled and fearful, but a heart filled with trust in God will be secure and at peace!

What is Cancer Anyway?

Lessons Learnt

- Our words have power if spoken in faith. Just as Jesus cursed the fig tree which bore no fruit, we can curse cancer cells and speak death over them.

- We need to guard our hearts against fear and put our trust in God.

Key Facts

- Cancerous cells multiply out of control and have no positive function in the body; in fact, they threaten the health of the body.

- There are more than a hundred distinctive forms of cancer.

- Not all forms of cancer are equally dangerous. Some are slow growing and treatable, whilst more dangerous cancers grow rapidly and spread more quickly.

Notes

1. American Cancer Society 2020. Questions People Ask About Cancer. Online article at URL:https://www.cancer.org/cancer/cancer-basics/questions-people-ask-about-cancer.html Accessed 2020-06-06

2. Mayo Clinic 2018. Cancer. Online article at URL:https://www.mayoclinic.org/diseases-conditions/cancer/symptoms-causes/syc-20370588 Accessed 2020-06-06

3. Shiel WC 2018. Medical Definition of Cancer. Online article at

URL:https://www.medicinenet.com/script/main/art.asp?articlekey=2580
Accessed 2020-06-0

Chapter 5

I Face My Goliath

My cardiologist, who was rather serious at the best of time, looked particularly glum as he scanned my results. As a keen swimmer and fitness fanatic, I would visit him once a year in the springtime for a stress ECG and a full battery of blood tests before I began my more rigorous summer exercise regime. Up to now the results had always been good, so I was expecting another thumbs-up.

He began with the good news that my heart was as fit as that of a healthy thirty-year old and that my blood tests were generally good. However, he said he was concerned that I had an elevated serum protein level. This could be for a variety of reasons; all fairly serious. I could have an auto-immune disease, HIV or Multiple Myeloma; a cancer of the bone marrow.

As I tried to process this rather alarming news, I returned to the pathology laboratory so that they could run further, more specific blood tests. They would conduct a HIV test and a serum electrophoresis test to get a better idea of what offending proteins were responsible for the elevated serum protein result.

A few days later I returned to the rooms in Nelspruit to hear the outcome of the results. It was bad news! My cardiologist was ninety-five percent sure that I had Multiple Myeloma (MM). He referred me to an oncologist and I would need to return yet again for further, more definitive tests. I remember sitting and waiting for my order in a fast food outlet and calling my beloved Desi to share this bad news which was too burdensome for me to carry alone. We both shed some tears over the phone as the horrible implications of the preliminary diagnosis began to sink in.

A Battery of Tests

This was to be a Thursday which I would sooner forget! We arrived at the hospital fairly early in the morning so that a variety of tests could be run. My first visit was to the X-ray department where they did a CT Scan of my thorax followed by a full set of X-rays of the rest of my body. This would show if there was evidence of multiple myeloma in my bones and would indicate the extent to which it had spread.

Following this, I went through the ordeal of having a bone marrow biopsy taken from my pelvis under only a local anaesthetic. The haematologist struggled to get a suitable sample for her microscopic examination and was only successful on about the fourth bone-crunching attempt. By this time, to my wife's alarm, the hospital bed was drenched in blood.

With this now done, we went to the oncology department for my first of many consultations with my oncologist. My wad of X-rays was under the arm. As we awaited our turn, I felt apprehensive and nervous like I imagine a criminal waiting in the dock for the judge's verdict might be. We observed the various patients moving in and out of the oncology department, wondering what their different stories might be. Some looked pretty healthy, whilst others looked pale and obviously ill. Most were able-bodied, whilst some shuffled along; a few were even wheeled in in wheelchairs. Questions crowded my mind: What would I look like six months from now? What did the future hold for me?

I Face My Goliath

Eventually our turn came and we were ushered into the oncologist's consulting room. She illuminated the X-rays and CT Scan for us and with the appropriate compassion and sensitivity, confirmed that I definitely had MM. She pointed out to us the various shaded areas in my skeletal system where myeloma was evident. There was a hole the size of a large coin through my pelvis. (This had probably been the site of the first plasmacytoma before the myeloma had spread to other areas). I now also had myeloma in my spine, neck and skull. Fortunately, none of my long bones in my arms or legs were affected. The news was simultaneously both shocking and unreal.

(Multiple myeloma is often only diagnosed when the vertebrae in a person's spine collapse or when an unexpected fracture of the limbs due to weakening and porosity of the bones is experienced. The reason it is called multiple myeloma is that this type of cancer usually spreads to multiple sites in the body before being detected.)

My doctor carefully explained to us the details of the disease called multiple myeloma or MM for short. MM is fairly treatable, but is regarded as an incurable disease. It is a cancer of the plasma cells in the bone marrow. Plasma cells produce the antibodies which protect us against disease. In the case of myeloma, cancerous plasma cells begin proliferating in the bone marrow, sometimes even damaging the bone structure, resulting in weakened areas and even holes. They crowd out the healthy plasma cells and produce large quantities of defective antibodies which result in high plasma protein levels. As a result, myeloma sufferers are usually immuno-compromised. Some go into acute kidney failure because of high levels of protein and calcium in the blood which compromise the liver and clog the kidneys.

(Again, some people are only diagnosed as having MM when they happen to go into acute kidney failure. Unfortunately, this happened to a friend of mine. Kidney failure is usually irreversible and the patient ends up needing to undergo dialysis on a regular basis until, if they are fortunate, they can receive a kidney transplant.)

I have much to be thankful for, in that I was diagnosed early, before any of these horrific complications of the disease set in. It did happen however, because I was proactive in monitoring my health on a regular basis. We take our vehicles in to be serviced every 15 000 km, and yet so many of us neglect monitoring our health and taking care of our bodies.

M-protein, standing for monoclonal protein (or para protein as it is referred to in some treatment centres) is a characteristic, defective antibody protein produced by cancerous plasma cells. Its level in the blood is a useful indicator of the presence and progress of the disease. My first, or baseline, M-protein reading when I was diagnosed, was 39 g/l. (A healthy person would have a reading of zero). Oncologists routinely monitor the full blood count of a patient including the liver and kidney functions as well as the M-protein reading.

A Word to Stand On

As my wife Desi and I listened to the verdict over my health, we sensed that I was facing a greater challenge than either of the previous two battles that I had fought against cancer. This was the monster! However, to keep our hearts from fear, the Holy Spirit immediately reminded us of the story of David fighting and killing the Philistine giant Goliath, which is recorded in *1 Samuel 17*. (Many of us have heard this Bible story from our childhood days but have never really applied it to our own battles in life. I would encourage you to read the story again with fresh ears and eyes.)

When the young boy David reached the battle lines with supplies for his older brothers, he heard the defiant challenges of Goliath the Philistine giant and witnessed how the army of Israel was paralysed with fear at his loud boasts. He was incensed at the man's arrogant defiance and asked, "*What will be done for the man who kills this Philistine and removes this disgrace from Israel? Who is this uncircumcised Philistine that he should defy the armies of the living God?*" **(1 Samuel 17:6)**

Word got to King Saul about David's comments and he summoned the young man. He was doubtful about David's ability to slay the giant, but David reassured him, saying "*Your servant has been keeping his father's sheep. When a lion or a bear came and carried off a sheep from the flock, I went after it, struck it and rescued the sheep from its mouth. When it turned on me, I seized it by its hair, struck it and killed it. Your servant has killed both the lion and the bear; this uncircumcised Philistine will be like one of them, because he has defied the armies of the living God. The LORD who delivered me from the paw of the lion and the paw of the bear will deliver me from the hand of this Philistine.*" **(1 Samuel 17:34-37)**

This last verse in particular spoke to us. Yes, the Lord had delivered me from both malignant melanoma and prostate cancer (the lion and the bear). Now, with God's help, I would surely defeat this Philistine called "Multiple Myeloma" with its loud boasts which was trying to instil fear in my heart. Through many of the battles which followed, I was able to stand on this word of Scripture.

Many will tell you that one of the keys to overcoming cancer is having a positive mind-set. However, I believe that more than positive thinking is required. We need to have a faith based on the words and promises of the Bible. In addition to this, it is also wonderful to have a prophetic word from God on which to base our hope and our faith. When Jesus was tempted by the Devil he said, "*It is written: 'Man does not live on bread alone, but on every word that comes from the mouth of God.'*"(**Matthew 4:4**) The Greek translation for "word" here, is *rhema* which is literally a 'spoken word.' A r*hema* word (or spoken word) from God quickens our faith since it becomes God's personal word to us.

We need a victorious mind-set and a conquering spirit like that of David to overcome cancer. He was aware that he was in covenant with the living God whereas Goliath was "uncircumcised" and had no covenant. If you are a believer, one of your covenant blessings from God is healing and health. Jesus called healing and deliverance from evil *"the children's bread"* or the food of God's children. *(See Mark 7:24-29)*

Back to our Bible story;

Instead of using Saul's sword and armour, David preferred to use his familiar weapon and went out against the giant with only his staff, five stones and a sling. The very first stone from his sling struck the giant's forehead and Goliath fell to the ground. Ironically, David used Goliath's own sword to cut off his head. We must not give way to fear, but in a fighting spirit "cut off the head" of cancer.

What about the other four stones? People love to speculate about these. Perhaps they were intended for the four other giants who David's mighty men killed in the course of time. *(See 2 Samuel 21:15-22)*. Spending time with David, they caught his victorious spirit and became giant killers themselves. If you or a loved one is facing the giant of cancer, it is my prayer that you too will become a giant killer!

Sharing the Burden of Bad News

When we are faced with a crisis or bear the burden of bad news, it is (or should be) instinctive for us to seek out those nearest and dearest to us. So, it was natural for Desi and me to immediately contact our children to inform them of my diagnosis. Although we shed some tears together over the phone, it was emotionally healing for me to experience their compassion and concern. As they say, "A burden shared is a burden halved." (Unfortunately, many people diagnosed with cancer keep it a secret and try to deal with the shock all on their own.)

Scripture encourages us saying: *Carry each other's burdens, and in this way, you will fulfil the law of Christ.* **(Galatians 6:2)**

Although they were sad and shocked, my three children, Stephen, Gina and Nicole, all committed to pray for me for my healing. A day later, my youngest, Nicole, who lives far across the seas in London, sent me these verses from Psalm 116 which I pondered and prayed through many times in the days to come:

> *I love the LORD, for he heard my voice; he heard my cry for mercy. Because he turned his ear to me, I will call on him as long as I live. The cords of death entangled me, the anguish of the grave came upon me; I was overcome by trouble and sorrow. Then I called on the name of the LORD: "O LORD, save me!" The LORD is gracious and righteous; our God is full of compassion. The LORD protects the simple-hearted; when I was in great need, he saved me. Be at rest once more, O my soul, for the LORD has been good to you. For you, O LORD, have delivered my soul from death, my eyes from tears, my feet from stumbling, that I may walk before the LORD in the land of the living.* —Psalm 116:1-9

As the senior pastor of Living Waters Church, I knew that sooner or later all our church members would hear the news that I had been diagnosed with cancer. Rather than having them hear the report second or third-hand, I decided it would be preferable to tell them the news myself in a carefully worded email which would also instil faith and hope. After all, what better group of people to share with than the community of faith? So, the very next Sunday, after our morning service, I called in all my leaders and told them my news. We had some quality time to share with one another and to pray together. Some shed tears of empathy and sorrow. Again, it was emotionally healing for Desi and me to be able to share our burden with those who loved and supported us. After this we "hit the send button" and informed the rest of the congregation via email.

Our church was and still is part of "The Christian Network" (TCN), a group of some two hundred churches across South Africa. At the time I was the Provincial Leader of TCN in Mpumalanga, so I contacted my colleagues in the TCN leadership group, as well as my regional leaders in Mpumalanga. My wife and I were bowled over by the amazing love and prayer support that we experienced from them throughout the months to come. At our next gathering, they laid hands upon me, anointed me with oil and prayed the prayer of faith for my healing. We are enjoined to do this in Scripture:

> *Is any one of you sick? He should call the elders of the church to pray over him and anoint him with oil in the name of the Lord. And the prayer offered in faith will make the sick person well; the Lord will raise him up. If he has sinned, he will be forgiven.* —James 5:14-15

It is tremendously reassuring to have men and women of God, people strong in faith, interceding for one. As Jesus said, there is power in agreement in prayer.

> *Again, I tell you that if two of you on earth agree about anything you ask for, it will be done for you by my Father in heaven. For where two or three come together in my name, there am I with them.* —Matthew 18:19-20

My brother and sister in the United States also joined the chorus of prayer together with my cousins in England. Eventually we truly had international support.

In the days to come various believers approached me and said they would like to pray with me for my healing. I admired their boldness and courage and appreciated their prayers. (I know that in some circumstances, especially for members of larger churches, this can become a bit much, but I believed the more prayers the better).

One thing that I did avoid however, was posting information on social media like Facebook. I did not want all and sundry to know the inside story of my battles and neither did I want any negative confessions or words of unbelief spoken out over my life. We can learn from Jesus' approach when he raised Jairus' little girl to life. He first put out the mourners, saying that the girl was not dead but only sleeping. I believe he didn't want or need a chorus of wailing and unbelief. Then he only took his closest disciples and the girl's parents into her room to witness her healing. What Jesus did want was the added faith of his disciples and the love and compassion of the parents for their daughter.

While Jesus was still speaking, some men came from the house of Jairus, the synagogue ruler. "Your daughter is dead," they said. "Why bother the teacher anymore?" Ignoring what they said, Jesus told the synagogue ruler, "Don't be afraid; just believe." He did not let anyone follow him except Peter, James and John the brother of James. When they came to the home of the synagogue ruler, Jesus saw a commotion, with people crying and wailing loudly. He went in and said to them, "Why all this commotion and wailing? The child is not dead but asleep." But they laughed at him. After he put them all out, he took the child's father and mother and the disciples who were with him, and went in where the child was. He took her by the hand and said to her, "Talithakoum!" (which means, "Little girl, I say to you, get up!"). Immediately the girl stood up and walked around (she was twelve years old). At this they were completely astonished. He gave strict orders not to let anyone know about this, and told them to give her something to eat. —Mark 5:35-43

We Need to be Real

I have spent some time talking about how I shared the burden of bad news because I believe that it is an important first step to prepare oneself for the battle which lies ahead. Many go into either denial or depression.

Those in denial are like the proverbial ostrich with its head in the sand. Because the news is bad they prefer to pretend that it's not true and try to put on a brave face and go on with life as if nothing has happened. Meanwhile, they are caving in on the inside. This is not faith; this is pretence. Faith faces the facts. Faith eventually triumphs despite the facts. Faith sometimes even changes the facts. (More about this later!)

The problem of denying or suppressing our emotions seems to be more prevalent amongst men. Many boys were taught during their childhood to suppress their emotions. They were taught to maintain a stiff British upper lip or that "cowboys don't cry." This approach to life is not Biblical at all. Jesus' second beatitude for us is, *Blessed are those who mourn, for they will be comforted.* **(Matthew 5:4)**

Yes, a cancer diagnosis often elicits a process of mourning and that is perfectly normal. So many things could potentially die. We mourn the fact that we may not be able to live out all our dreams or grow old together as husband and wife etc.

The opposite extreme to denial, is when people are so shocked and impacted by the doctor's verdict that they have cancer, that they see it almost as a death sentence. As a result, they end up being emotional wrecks wallowing in self-pity or in the depths of depression. This is definitely not a good starting point if you are about to wage a war of life and death.

We should not be controlled by our emotions, but rather manage and adjust them to meet the challenge. Unruly emotions impacted by fear or self-pity could result in defeat before the battle really begins, so our spirits under the control of the Holy Spirit must ultimately rule over our souls. David was very aware of what was going on in his soul and took charge over unruly emotions:

Why are you downcast, O my soul? Why so disturbed within me? Put your hope in God, for I will yet praise him, my Savior and my God...
—Psalm 42:5-6

One positive outcome of a cancer diagnosis is that it clarifies for us the nature of the enemy we face. The advice of a good army general would be, "know your enemy." Once we know the enemy we can begin preparing our hearts to meet the challenge. My approach of sharing the burden with others and eliciting prayer support helped me to begin processing my emotions and yes, I did shed some tears, but that was only for a season. We are emotional and social beings and the compassion and comfort of others will help us to cope and ultimately conquer. That is why God's family, the church is taught to:

Rejoice with those who rejoice; mourn with those who mourn. —Romans 12:15

Our hero David, the great warrior and giant slayer, was in touch with his emotions and often wept. Many of his

47

Psalms are laments. Here is one example which spoke to me because it refers to bone pain which many cancer patients suffer:

> *O LORD, do not rebuke me in your anger or discipline me in your wrath. Be merciful to me, LORD, for I am faint; O LORD, heal me, for my bones are in agony. My soul is in anguish. How long, O LORD, how long? Turn, O LORD, and deliver me; save me because of your unfailing love. No one remembers you when he is dead. Who praises you from the grave? I am worn out from groaning; all night long I flood my bed with weeping and drench my couch with tears.* —Psalm 6:1-6

After an emotional catharsis like this, David would invariably pull himself together and take courage. As a result, many of his laments end on a positive, hopeful note.

So, what is the bottom line? What am I trying to say? I'm campaigning for a balanced emotional response to the challenge of cancer which avoids the two unhealthy extremes of denial or emotionalism. Since we are emotional beings we should expect that our emotions will push to the surface occasionally. When they do, it is healthy to acknowledge them and to process them. However, we must not dwell on them or allow them to unduly dictate our response. Our faith in God must remain our anchor during the storms of life.

> *We have this hope as an anchor for the soul, firm and secure. It enters the inner sanctuary behind the curtain, where Jesus, who went before us, has entered on our behalf. He has become a high priest forever, in the order of Melchizedek.*
> —Hebrews 6:19-20

Lessons Learnt

- More than positive thinking is required when we face spiritual battles; we need to have a faith based on the words and promises of the Bible.

- It is also wonderful to have a specific, prophetic word from God on which to base our hope and our faith.

- If you are a believer in Christ, one of your covenant blessings from God is healing and health.

- It is emotionally healing for us to share our bad news with those close to us and to experience their compassion and concern.

- Be careful with whom you share your news to avoid any negative confessions or words of unbelief being spoken out over your life.

- Processing one's emotions is an important first step to prepare oneself for the battle which lies ahead.

- A cancer diagnosis clarifies for us the nature of the enemy we face. Once we know the enemy we can begin preparing our hearts to meet the challenge.

- Our spirits under the control of the Holy Spirit, must ultimately rule over our souls.

- We need a balanced emotional response to the challenge of cancer which avoids the two unhealthy extremes of denial or emotionalism.

Key Facts

- As we get older, we should be pro-active in monitoring our health regularly. This is especially important for the early detection of cancer.

Chapter 6

Venturing into the Unknown

Life is a series of new beginnings. Like our first day at "big school", we begin at the bottom and gradually progress to the top. Eventually we occupy the privileged position of being a senior, only to find that the very next year we have to begin again as a junior in "high school" and must negotiate the challenges of initiation before we can progress. And so, the cycles go on...

For those diagnosed with cancer and needing chemotherapy, the first day in the "chemo room" is another such challenging new beginning, another such rite of passage if you like. Chemotherapy is a weighty word which carries with it many perceptions. As a result, there is a certain amount of fear that accompanies you as you venture into this new, unknown territory. You wonder if you will be able to handle the needles and the side-effects. You've heard of people being nauseous for days, throwing up, having sores in their mouths and of course you've seen pale, bald-headed people without any eyebrows who are undergoing the ravages of chemotherapy.

Far from being a hostile environment, I soon found the chemo room to be a kind of clubhouse for cancer comrades. The chemo sister was kind and reassuring and an expert at finding a vein for her needle with a minimum amount of pain or fuss. There was also a great sense of camaraderie amongst the patients who swapped stories about the rigors of their particular brand of cancer and chemo. Although we were undergoing different treatments, we were all somehow in the same boat. (Often, an entirely different combination of drugs is used for treating a different class of cancer).

I needed a weekly infusion of two drugs and a sub-cutaneous injection of a third. I had elected to have my treatment on a Monday, so I made weekly trips through to the city of Nelspruit. There were others who also regularly had treatments on that day and I soon became part of the "Monday crowd." Once more, like in the past, I was care-ful not to "Bible bash" any of the other patients, but it wasn't long before a number found out that I was a pastor and began asking me questions. It was an excellent oppor-tunity to offer comfort and encouragement.

From time to time, newbies joined the group. It was easy to pick them out. They were a bit wide-eyed, fearful and obviously unfamiliar with the territory. Some had re-cently been diagnosed with cancer and were still in some shock. The veterans in the group always made a point of reassuring them and making them feel at home and the chemo sister would take extra care of them as she put up their first drip.

Deadly Poison

Cancer cells generally multiply at a much faster rate than normal cells, so traditional chemotherapy drugs act by halt-ing or slowing down cell division in the body. This is designed to compromise the progress of the cancer selec-tively, but it invariably also impacts other healthy, fast-growing cells in the body.

Rapid cell division takes place in our bone marrow in order to produce new blood cells. Red blood cells (eryth-rocytes) survive for about 115 days before needing replacement, whilst white blood cells (leucocytes) and platelets (thrombocytes) survive for only a couple of days. Chemotherapy drugs negatively impact the production of blood cells by slowing down cell replication in the bone marrow. As a result, the patient can become anaemic (having a low red blood cell count and a low haemoglobin reading) and may also suffer leucopoenia (having a low white blood cell count) which may result in reduced immunity. A low platelet count predisposes the patient to the danger of bleeding. (MM patients also have frequent liver and kidney function tests as well as serum electrophoresis to monitor M-protein and/or light chain serum proteins).

To make sure that the dosage of the chemotherapy drugs is not having excessively negative effects, a full blood count is usually done before administering the next cycle of chemo. One soon becomes familiar with being poked with needles for these regular blood tests. Cancer is definitely not for sissies!

Other organs and tissues in the body also have rapidly dividing cells which are unfortunately also negatively impacted by chemotherapy drugs. These include our hair follicles (that is why some drugs cause hair loss) and the epithelial layers of our alimentary canal/gastro intestinal tract (that is why we may develop ulcers in the mouth or suffer nausea, constipation or diarrhoea.) One area of the brain also has rapidly dividing cells and may be adversely affected. People talk about having "chemo brain" which can cause forgetfulness.

From the above we can see that, since these drugs affect so many areas of our bodies and slow down cell division, being treated with them is somewhat like drinking deadly poison.

Targeted Drugs

Fortunately, medical science is continually advancing and more effective, less-damaging drugs are continually being discovered and developed. There have been great advances in the treatment of multiple myeloma and as a result the average life expectancy of patients receiving treatment has increased substantially.

A class of drugs known as proteasome inhibitors has proved to be very effective in the treatment of MM. They are much more targeted in their action, killing principally cancer cells and they generally have fewer side-effects than classical chemotherapy drugs.

For those who want to know…

Proteasomes are tiny, barrel shaped structures found in all cells. Their job is to rid the cell of mis-folded, "used", and non-functional proteins like a garbage disposal. Once these proteins are broken up, the cell can then use them to make new proteins that it might need… Although normal cells make proteins, so do cancerous plasma cells - but they make much larger amounts of useless, inef-fective protein. When a proteasome inhibitor stops this protein "recycling," it allows the protein to build up until it blows the cell up. The cell dies of built-up bad, accumulated waste. (Ahlstrom 2016)

There are currently three proteasome inhibitors that are used for multiple myeloma (MM) treat-ment: Velcade (bortezomib), Kyprolis (carfil-zomib), and Ninlaro (ixazomib). (Multiple Myeloma Research Foundation 2017)

Several other drugs are still under development so there is a growing list of treatment options for MM sufferers. There are also some very exciting developments in using immunological treatments.

My Weekly Cocktail

During the first phase of my treatment (the induction phase), I was put on a drug cocktail abbreviated as:

BOR/DEX/CYCLO. (Not the kind of cocktail you'd like to order from the bar during "happy hour"!)

BOR stands for Bortezomib – one of the targeted drugs with few side-effects.

DEX stands for Dexamethasone – a corticosteroid. It is notorious for having a variety of side-effects. (Jenny Ahlstrom, an MM patient and founder of The Myeloma Crowd even wrote a song about her tumultuous relationship with Dex)[3].

CYCLO stands for Cyclophosphamide – a classical chemotherapy drug with its own set of potential side-effects.

This combination of drugs is fairly effective, but is also expensive, so we prayed that our medical aid/insurance would approve the treatment. My oncologist wrote a motivation letter and thankfully approval was quickly granted.

Excellent Progress with Minimal Side-Effects

As I mentioned earlier, I started treatment with a baseline M-protein score of 39. In the first month it dropped to 13; exactly one-third of what it had been. (Which occasioned some loud Hallelujahs!). The following month I was down to 7, then to 5, then to 4. This is apparently a typical graph one can expect.

I was very aware that I was being carried in prayer by my family, our church congregation and prayer warriors around the world as they bound cancer and loosed healing over my life.

Jesus said, *I tell you the truth, whatever you bind on earth will be bound in heaven, and whatever you loose on earth will be loosed in heaven. Again, I tell you that if two of you on earth agree about anything you ask for, it will be done for you by my Father in heaven.* **(Matthew 18:18-19)**

Thankfully I got right down to zero in 6 months – just before the second phase of my treatment which was my stem cell transplant.

Jesus also said an interesting thing before He returned to heaven:

> **...these signs will accompany those who believe: In my name they will drive out demons; they will speak in new tongues; they will pick up snakes with their hands; and when they drink deadly poison, it will not hurt them at all; they will place their hands on sick people, and they will get well."** — Mark 16:17-18

Did you get the one about deadly poison? *...when they drink deadly poison, it will not hurt them at all...*

As a believer I took this verse literally as applying to me. I would pray before my chemo treatments that the drugs would go straight to target and kill cancer cells but cause minimal damage to healthy cells and have minimal side-effects. I prayed that, as I was infused with what could be regarded as deadly poison, it would not harm me at all. Now you can berate me for being a literalist, but my testimony is that I have experienced almost zero side-effects whilst receiving chemo over the past three years.

A Prayer to Pray

Jesus, you said that believers could drink even deadly poison and it would not harm them. I believe in you and I ask that as I receive my chemo today it will not harm any healthy cells in my body but that it will go straight to target and kill only cancer cells. I speak death to cancer and life to my body in your mighty name. Amen.

During my regular consultations with my oncologist she would rattle off a list of questions about my condition to which I would invariably respond in the negative:

"Do you have sores in your mouth?"

"No!"

"Are you suffering from constipation or diarrhoea?"

"No!"

"Are you experiencing any pain when I press on your spine?"

"No!"

She would also check my lungs using her stethoscope - they were invariably clear. I have never thrown up, not even when I went through the challenging ordeal of a stem cell transplant which included high-dose chemotherapy. (More about this later).

About the only side-effect I did experience was that on Mondays and Tuesdays I was full of energy as a result of having had steroids. The students at our Bible College who met on a Monday night, would comment about how energetic and humorous I was. I was so hyped up that I had to take a sleeping tablet on Monday nights. On Tuesday mornings I would have a vigorous exercise session to work off some of the energy and make good use of the steroids in order to put on some muscle.

In those first six months, in addition to my normal pastoral duties, I also did major renovations to our church buildings. I completely redecorated the bathrooms, our fellowship hall and did some necessary upgrades in our youth hall. Unlike many others, I enjoyed a pretty productive relationship with Dex!

Lessons Learnt

- Receiving treatment for cancer is often an opportunity to forge new friendships with people who are in the same boat.

- We can pray in faith that the drugs with which we are being treated will be effective and kill cancer cells whilst having minimal side-effects.

Key Facts

- Often, an entirely different combination of drugs is used for treating a different class of cancer.

- Chemotherapy drugs slow down cell division in the body. This is designed to compromise the progress of the cancer selectively, but it invariably also impacts other healthy, rapidly dividing cells in the body.

- In order to make sure that the dosage of the chemotherapy drugs is not having excessively negative effects, a full blood count is usually done before administering the next cycle of chemo.

- Targeted drugs principally kill cancer cells and they generally have fewer side-effects than classical chemotherapy drugs.

- A combination or "cocktail" of drugs is often used to treat cancer.

Notes:

1. Ahlstrom J 2016. How Proteasome Inhibitors Work. Online article at

    URL:https://www.myelomacrowd.org/myeloma-101-proteasome-inhibitors-work/ Accessed 2020-06-20

2. Multiple Myeloma Research Foundation 2017. Proteasome Inhibitors. Online article at URL:https://themmrf.org/uncategorized/proteasome-inhibitors/ Accessed 2020-06-20

3. Ahlstrom J 2016. I Will Say Goodbye: A Song. Online article at URL:https://www.myelomacrowd.org/songs-life-heartfelt-song-dex/ Accessed 2020-06-22

CHAPTER 7

BOOT CAMP

The "induction" phase of my treatment had involved four cycles of fairly intensive chemotherapy. This had been designed to bring the cancer under control and had done just that. It had brought with it some anticipated challenges, but my response to the drugs had been good, my M-protein count having dropped from 39 to 4. Now followed what was known as the "consolidation" phase. During this phase I was to undergo an autologous stem cell transplant at Alberts Cellular Therapy Clinic (ACT Clinic) in Pretoria, the capital city of South Africa. The ACT Clinic at Netcare Hospital, Pretoria East is probably the most advanced and prestigious unit of its kind on the continent of Africa. I would be under the care of a clinical haematologist and a whole team of physicians and nurses during this phase.

Prior to the consolidation phase, I was granted a well-deserved holiday of a full month of respite from chemotherapy in order to cleanse my system of the drugs and to prepare myself for my transplant. My oncologist was aware that I had been exercising regularly during my induction and she urged me to continue doing so. She said it would be to my advantage if I was super fit as I faced the challenge of having a stem cell transplant.

This was enough motivation for me to increase the intensity of my exercise program. During that month, which was somewhat like a personal boot camp for me, I swam a mile three times a week in the blue waters of the Sabie Country Club swimming pool. In the early mornings I had the pool all to myself and I would pray out loud as I did stretch exercises between splits of different strokes and kicks.

On three other days of the week I would don my cycling gear and head off into the forests around Sabie on my mountain bike. There is nothing as exhilarating as whizzing down a single track through a pine forest, stopping for a breather at a waterfall, or taking in the view from the top of a mountain. It was an excellent time to prepare myself, not only physically, but also spiritually, and I had a very real sense of the presence of God. Father would whisper in my spirit, *"I am with you my son."* What reassuring words!

Many people regard a casual stroll around the block as exercise. However, I quickly realised that something more challenging than this would be necessary if I was going to reap the benefits of exercise.

You might be wondering why I consider exercise to be so important in the fight against cancer. It is obvious that simply getting the blood circulating and increasing the metabolic rate has the advantage of helping one's body eradicate the toxins and breakdown products of the chemo. There's also nothing like a bit of healthy sweat to aid the process! I would also recommend drinking copious amounts of water to assist the liver and kidneys in this detox process. MM patients, in particular, need to keep their kidneys as healthy as possible and avoid renal failure at all costs.

Many cancer sufferers being treated with chemo are anaemic and have to do as much as they can by means of diet and exercise to counteract this. The good news is that regular, vigorous aerobic exercise, which maintains an elevated pulse rate for more than 15 minutes, helps stimulate red blood cell production and increases one's haemoglobin level.

Aerobic exercise can alter the number of red blood cells in several ways. Red blood cells carry oxygen and carbon dioxide through the bloodstream. In general, endurance training increases the number of red blood cells. (Miller 2020)

Exercise training can increase total Hb and red cell mass, which enhances oxygen-carrying capacity. The possible underlying mechanisms are proposed to come mainly from bone marrow, including stimulated erythropoiesis with hyperplasia of the hematopoietic bone marrow... (Hu and Lin 2012)

Ensuring that you are eating a healthy, iron rich diet also aids the process. During my personal boot camp, I ate plenty of green vegetables rich in iron like spinach, kale, broccoli and beans as well as animal protein which contains haem iron, like red meat, liver, fish etc. I also ate plenty of fruit, including vitamin C rich fruits like oranges, grapefruit and naartjies. At the end of my time of preparation my blood results were excellent. Both my red blood cell and white blood cell counts were well into the normal range and my haemoglobin level was remarkably good.

Putting Plans in Place

My wife and I would need to be in the vicinity of Pretoria for nearly two months so it was necessary for us to make some detailed plans regarding the ministry of our church during our absence. Fortunately, I had a team of very understanding and willing leaders and Hein, my capable young associate pastor. They were all ready to step up to the challenge of preaching and running the services.

We decided to embark on a ten-week series on the ten commandments which would maintain a sense of direction and cohesion during my absence. Pastor Leonard Stone, the author of the series, was the national leader of TCN (our network of churches) and he undertook to send a couple of his men from Maranatha Community Church in Kempton Park to preach two of the ten sessions; the rest would be handled by local talent. Liz, my personal assistant, would be well able to "hold fort" at the church office and to keep the administrative wheels turning. A couple of my leaders were part of our Bible College and they undertook to facilitate the sessions in my absence.

We would have to leave our house unattended for the period. I remember doing odd jobs around the house, like checking outside lights and making sure that the burglar alarm was working properly. Much to our sorrow, our two old Dachshunds had died toward the end of the previous year, but this meant there was not the added complication of needing to have a house-sitter to look after our dogs. We trusted the Lord to look after our property in our absence.

Packing for Pretoria

Information about exactly what I was in for was rather sketchy. I had been given a provisional time table listing some of the key events, but the dates were not definite. I was aware that the first month would involve stimulating the production of stem cells and then harvesting them. During the next month I would be going into an isolation ward for at least three weeks when they would perform my stem cell transplant. Following the transplant, I would remain in isolation until the transplant had "grafted" and my blood counts returned to acceptable levels.

We were also a bit unclear on what to pack for the isolation ward. I had been told that in my room in Ward 20, I would have my own bathroom, Lazyboy armchair, TV, desk and bar fridge. It all sounded quite luxurious and I wondered if it was going to be like a three-week holiday. (Ha ha!) I anticipated having oodles of time at my disposal and decided to make the most of it, so I packed a number of books and magazines, my guitar, my laptop and tablet and things to keep me occupied. I even included a plastic step to enable me to continue my exercise program. The bottom line was that I ended up taking along far too much stuff. Desi did a great job of packing my clothes, various permissible foodstuffs and some goodies to remind me that I was loved.

Eventually the day of our departure arrived and we headed to my mother in law's retirement home in Benoni. This was to be my base of operations during the times I was not hospitalised and Desi's base for the duration of the time. A big challenge at the time and something which delayed my transplant by a week was the fact that the costly procedure had not yet been authorised by my Medical Aid. A body called the South African Oncology Consortium (SAOC) had to meet to deliberate whether I was a worthy candidate for the procedure. If they gave the green light, my Medical Aid Society would be honour-bound to meet the obligation to fund the transplant. The problem was that the SAOC had not met for some time as some of its members had been on leave, so we were left anxiously kicking our heels in Benoni for a week. Eventually the approval came through and we were off to Pretoria for my pre-transplant tests.

Pre-Screening

A stem cell transplant is quite a physically challenging medical procedure even for the healthiest individual, so I was subjected to a whole range of tests before finally being accepted. (One kind of gets the impression that it's going to be a case of the survival of the fittest.)

They tested nearly everything you could think of – from the routine to the obscure. They did the routine blood tests, but also included detailed liver and kidney function tests. My blood was also tested for various diseases like malaria, hepatitis and HIV amongst others. Then I also had an ECG, a chest X-ray, a heart sonar and a lung capacity test.

I was eventually deemed fit enough to endure the rigours of a transplant, so I was given the thumbs-up and the treatment process began.

Lessons Learnt

- Fighting cancer is as much a spiritual battle as it is a physical one and we need to be prepared and strengthened on both fronts.

Key Facts

- Exercise increases blood circulation, stimulates the metabolism and helps the body to detox.

- Aerobic and anaerobic exercise can help alleviate anaemia by stimulating red blood cell production and raising the haemoglobin level in the blood.

- A stem cell transplant is a physically challenging medical procedure even for the healthiest individual.

Notes

1. Miller J 2020. Does Exercise Increase Red Blood Cells? Online article at URL: https://www.livestrong.com/article/534560-does-exercise-increase-red-blood-cells/ Accessed 2020-06-27

2. Hu M and Lin W 2012. Effects of exercise training on red blood cell production: implications for ane-

mia. ActaHaematol. 127(3):156-64. Online article at URL: https://pubmed.ncbi.nlm.nih.gov/22301865/ Accessed 2020-06-27

Chapter 8

Tested by Fire

God is excellent, perfect, holy and majestic... *God is light; in him there is no darkness at all.* (*1 John 1:5*) *He is the Rock; His deeds are perfect. Everything He does is just and fair. He is a faithful God who does no wrong; how just and upright He is!* (*Deuteronomy 32:4 NLT*)

It seems that this excellent God has high standards of quality which He insists on maintaining. Therefore, before we can progress to the next level in our walk of faith, we will have to pass a test or two. Consequently, we are forewarned in Scripture concerning the testing and refining of our faith:

> **In this you greatly rejoice, though now for a little while you may have had to suffer grief in all kinds of trials. These have come so that your faith—of greater worth than gold, which perishes even though refined by fire—may be proved genuine and may result in praise, glory and honor when** ***Jesus Christ is revealed.*** —1 Peter 1:6-7

The tests will come sooner or later. Fortunately, God also promises not to test us beyond our strength and always to provide a way out. (*See 1 Corinthians 10:13*)

Mobilisation

One of the doctors who was part of the team at ACT Clinic carefully explained to Desi and me what the first phase of the transplant, known as "mobilisation" would entail.

Our bone marrow is a sponge-like matrix in the core of all our bones. Hematopoietic stem cells located in this spongy matrix can differentiate into a variety of specialised cells which are the precursors of our different classes of blood cells. During mobilisation I would be treated with a chemotherapy drug which would break down this spongy matrix and free or "mobilise" the stem cells so that they would begin to circulate in the peripheral blood.

To stimulate the stem cells to multiply, I would be injected for several days with a hormone known as Neupogen. My blood would be monitored regularly and once there were sufficient stem cells ($CD34^+$ cells) circulating, they would be harvested and kept in cryogenic storage until the day of my transplant. This is what happens in what is known as an "autologous stem cell transplant" (where the donor and the recipient are the same person). This took place in my case.

However, if it were deemed unlikely that they would be able to harvest healthy stem cells from a patient, a suitable, matching bone marrow donor would need to be found. The donor would have to go through a similar mobilisation process and his/her stem cells would be harvested. The harvested stem cells would then be transplanted into the patient. This is known as an "allogenic stem cell transplant" (where the donor and the recipient are different individuals).

Following the successful harvesting of my stem cells I would be given a week's break and then would follow the more challenging transplant phase during which I would be confined to an isolation ward.

Once this briefing was over, I was settled into my first room in the isolation ward. I would only occupy it for three days whilst I had my first two doses of chemo designed to break down the bone marrow matrix. Desi and I were given the run-down on the protocols designed to maintain sterility in Ward 20. If she wished to visit me, she would need to wear a sterile gown, a mask and gloves and cover her shoes. Only two nurses would attend to me: one during the day shift and one at night. They too would wear all the gear needed to maintain sterility.

Isolation of the patient together with these stringent sterility procedures is necessary because those who have been treated with high-dose chemotherapy have very low white blood cell counts and thus have drastically reduced immunity. The rooms are kept sparkling clean and have no opening windows. They are kept under positive pressure with sterile filtered air from a specialist air conditioning plant.

Slammed by a Six-Pack

Fairly late in the afternoon of the next day I was taken in a wheelchair to the chemo room on the third floor of the ACT Clinic. It is an all-glass penthouse room with beautiful vistas of the surrounding suburbs of Pretoria. I was to receive the drug Etoposide which tends to crystallise fairly quickly. To avoid this, I would be infused with six separate sachets of the drug rather than one large sachet. Whilst one was being run rapidly intravenously, the next sachet would be prepared. I joked with the nursing sister about her 'slamming me with a six-pack!'

The fast infusion could apparently be quite a shock to my system, so I was linked up to a heart monitor and my blood pressure was also monitored continuously throughout the process. The drug also had the notorious reputation of causing hair loss about a fortnight after being administered. (True to form, it was exactly two weeks to the day when large clumps of my hair began to fall out).

As these drips were quickly run into my arm, I began to feel faint and dizzy and the room began to spin. To top it all a storm began to brew and lightning flashed all around the penthouse chemo room. It was like a spectacular, psychedelic light show, quite a surreal experience that I will never forget. Fortunately, I had my son Stephen with me as a stabilising influence.

A Hellish Night

I felt okay by the time I was returned to my room in the isolation ward, but that night I had a rare but quite severe reaction to the drug. I began to run a fever and rigors set in. One minute I felt hot and the next I was shivering with my teeth chattering.

I prayed up a storm, taking authority over the fever and claiming the promise that, should I drink even deadly poison it would not harm me. My male nurse, who had been nicknamed "Superman" by the other staff, was quite alarmed and said that if my temperature rose any further, he would have to follow protocol and transfer me to the Intensive Care Unit. I assured him all would be well since I was praying to the Living God and my God would surely answer. He too was a believer and agreed to stand in faith with me.

It is a wonderful privilege to be able to call on a living, loving God in the midst of a crisis. In fact, we are encouraged to do this: ...*call upon me in the day of trouble; I will deliver you, and you will honor me.* **(Psalm 50:15)**

When I ran out of words to pray in English, I continued praying in other tongues. I am so thankful that in times of weakness or when I run out of my human resources, I can call on my helper – the Holy Spirit. As I prayed in an unknown language, I sensed that the Holy Spirit was interceding for me just as the following Scripture indicates:

> *...the Spirit helps us in our weakness. We do not know what we ought to pray for, but the Spirit himself intercedes for us with groans that words*

cannot express. And he who searches our hearts knows the mind of the Spirit, because the Spirit intercedes for the saints in accordance with God's will. —Rom 8:26-27

It was a long, hard fight for some four to five hours, but eventually my temperature began to return to normal and the rigors passed. Superman was suitably relieved and I was thankful that he had not transferred me to ICU.

As if all of this had not been enough, in the early hours of the following morning there was another heavy thunderstorm. This time the storm was accompanied by a heavy downpour of rain. I began to hear dripping in my room and when I put on a light, I noticed that the floor was a couple of centimetres deep in water. I rang for help and Superman eventually managed to mop things up using several hospital blankets.

This Scripture seemed to encapsulate the kind of night that I had just been through:

When you pass through deep waters, I will be with you; your troubles will not overwhelm you. When you pass through fire, you will not be burned; the hard trials that come will not hurt you. —Isa 43:2 GNB

The following day I had to be infused with a further six sachets of Etoposide, but this time the overseeing doctor took some extra precautions to prevent the unusual shock reaction to the drug which I had experienced. I was heavily sedated whilst on the drip and struggled to keep my eyes open. All went well and after spending another night under observation in the isolation ward I was pleased to be allowed to go home for some time to my base in Benoni.

Fighting Infection

In a couple of days, I began self-injecting with the hormone Neupogen at 6am every morning; this would stimulate stem cell production. If all went well, I would be able to stay at home providing I continually monitored my temperature and made several visits to the hospital to have my blood tested.

All went well for about a week and then I noticed that I was running a slight fever. My temperature began to climb, but for a while I kept it a secret from my wife and began to fight it on my own. It was amazing to me how, in the hour of trouble, the Holy Spirit reminded me of just about every healing Scripture in the Bible. I quoted these as I prayed and rebuked the Evil One and his sickness, determined not to accept his "package" without a fight. I claimed the promises of the Word of God and spoke out healing over my body.

A Prayer for Healing

Father God, I thank you that you introduced yourself to us as Jehovah Rophe, the Lord our healer. I come to you now, my Healer, in the name of your Son Jesus who took up our infirmities and who carried our diseases and by whose stripes we are healed. I ask that you touch me and heal me now. Drive out this infirmity and sickness from my body I pray. May your Holy Spirit brood over me and impart life and health to my body. I thank you that you forgive all my sins and heal all of my diseases in the name of Jesus. Amen.

To cool myself off I took a couple of cold showers. Eventually my wife became aware of what was going on and she joined me in the fight. We agreed in prayer as she sponged me with water and fanned me in an attempt to cool me. I again began to experience rigors; my teeth began chattering and I experienced difficulty breathing. Having given birth to our three children, Desi had experienced what was involved in labour and instructed me on how to relax and to breathe intentionally. My temperature peaked at around 39.7⁰C

After several hours my temperature began to return to normal and, following the fight, I had a fairly restful night of sleep. However, during the following day my temperature again began to climb. We decided that it was time to be obedient and follow my doctor's guidelines. Because it was a weekend, I called the doctor on emergency duty and was instructed to make haste and get to the hospital.

I was confined to a bed in Ward 2 (a general cancer ward) and, after confirming that I had a lung infection, they put me on a suitable antibiotic. In a couple of days, the infection was a thing of the past. The medical staffers were amazed at how quickly I recovered from the infection. I believe that this was because of the prayer foundation which had already been laid. This is another confirmation to me that there is no conflict between exercising faith and receiving medication. We should take medication in faith that it will be effective and accomplish what it is intended to do as quickly as possible.

We should never underestimate the power and the compassion of our God. David had a revelation of both: *One thing God has spoken, two things have I heard: that you, O God, are strong, and that you, O Lord, are loving... (Psa 62:11-12)*

The church back home in Sabie was also praying for my recovery. We should never underestimate the power of prayer:

...The prayer of a righteous man is powerful and effective. Elijah was a man just like us. He prayed earnestly that it would not rain, and it did not rain on the land for three and a half years. Again he prayed, and the heavens gave rain, and the earth produced its crops. —James 5:16-18

The Wonders of Ward 2

Hospital wards can be interesting places with their ups and downs and one has to be both resilient and have a sense of humour in order to survive. I tried to make the most of my confinement and to see the funny side in some of the things that happened, whilst some other events were of such a serious nature that there was just nothing humorous about them.

There were four beds in my room in Ward 2 and it was a good opportunity to make friends of other patients who were also fighting cancer.

Dazed and Confused

I soon made good friends with another man who, like me, had multiple myeloma and was undergoing a stem cell transplant. He was a little ahead of me in the scheme of things and also had to return to hospital because of an infection. His stem cells reached a suitable level a couple of days ahead of mine and he was taken through for them to be harvested. He returned some hours later and was very upbeat about the fact that they had been able to harvest enough cells for several transplants.

Unfortunately, they had not been able to find suitable veins in his arms for the harvesting procedure so they had cut into a major vein in his thigh. For some reason, he still had a tube attached to his thigh when he returned. That night he became a bit confused and got out of his bed and went wandering around. He fell down in the corner of our room and somehow dislodged the tube still attached to his thigh. There was soon blood everywhere. I rang the emergency bell for the nurse and they were soon on the scene trying to calm down my dazed friend and to sort out the chaos.

They put him back in his bed and raised the sides to stop him from wandering. Some hours later he again tried to leave his bed and I had to call the sister on duty to help. The whole event was a sobering reminder that we were not here playing games, but that life and death issues were at stake. I wondered what my harvesting experience would be like. Would they find suitable veins in my arms or would a similar surgical procedure be necessary for them to draw sufficient blood for their harvesting machine? Would I also end up dazed and confused as my friend had been?

Lewis Takes on the Ladies

A new patient, Lewis, (not his real name) was admitted and the rest of us in the room greeted him warmly. We only received a grunt in reply. He clearly didn't want to talk, so we left him to himself. They put up some drips and began treating him with chemo. The nurses were also finding it difficult to get him to communicate with them or to cooperate. However, sometime after midnight, when we were all fast asleep, he suddenly found his voice. He bellowed that he'd had enough and began demanding that they discharge him from the hospital immediately.

When the nurse on duty in our room could not convince him to calm down, she called the senior sister in charge of the ward. Eventually there were three female staff members trying to sort him out. He demanded that they call his doctor, but they made it clear that this was not possible in the early hours of the morning. Undauntedly he demanded that they call the matron of the hospital. Again, they insisted that this was not in line with hospital proto-col. The whole encounter was quite amusing. I have a sneaky feeling that they eventually laced his drip with a strong tranquiliser because he quickly lost steam and fell asleep. He should have thought twice about challenging authority in a matriarchal society!

Things Can Get Noisy

From the above two incidents you can see that it would be an understatement to say that I was not enjoying very rest-ful nights of sleep.

Something else took place routinely every night when I had just dozed off – the water jugs arrived! A staff mem-ber would wheel a cart packed full of jugs of drinking wa-ter down the main passage. I wouldn't care, but it sounded as if the cart had square wheels which caused all the jugs to jingle against each other and make a huge cacophony. I investigated the offending cart one morning and found that the wheels were in fact round, but that they were of old battle-scarred solid rubber – small wonder that the whole contraption kicked up such a noise!

Ward 2 was the general oncology ward and dealt with many immune-suppressed cancer patients so they also maintained strict sterility protocols (although not as strict as those of Ward 20 – the isolation ward.) Whenever a patient vacated a bed the staff would go through a rigorous procedure of cleaning and sterilising the bed and entire surrounding area. This was quite noisy in itself, but one night two of the nursing staff decided to take the sterility protocols to the next level.

Whilst the three of us patients left in the room tried to get some sleep, they completely dismantled the vacant hospital bed. They then sterilised each component and reassembled the bed piece-by-piece. Although the nurses spoke in hushed tones I'm afraid the whole procedure proved to be a bit of a nightmare for me.

The Day of Nine Needles

During any hospital stay one is invariably coupled up to an intravenous drip. Drips tend to have a lifespan of only a few days before they block or start leaking, then another suitable vein has to be found. The whole process of the nursing sister finding a vein and inserting a needle can be quite painful and I found that some staffers were much better than others at the task.

Another thing takes place daily with cancer patients; a nurse (phlebotomist) from the pathology lab arrives at around 4am to draw blood for various tests. This is so that the results will already be available when the doctors do their rounds at around 8am. If the phlebotomist fails to locate a suitable vein in three attempts, he/she has to call a colleague to have a go.

On one particular day I ended up like a proverbial pin cushion; I counted that I'd had nine needles thrust into my veins with several of them failing to hit target. I titled this record in my diary as "The Day of Nine Needles".

Dear reader, please realise that cancer is not for sissies! If you are to survive the challenges of chemotherapy and hospital wards, you have to overcome the fear of needles and you need to be resilient. Think of yourself as "the Ultimate Survivor."

Abundant Harvest

The day of nine needles also turned out to be a day of celebration. After the phlebotomists finally managed to draw blood samples for testing, the results came back showing that my stem cell count ($CD34^+$ count) had soared to a "massive high" (to use my doctor's terminology) and was definitely at a suitable level for me to undergo "apheresis".

In medical jargon, apheresis refers to a technique by which a particular substance or component is removed from the blood and the main volume is then returned to the body. In my case this would mean the removal of stem cells from my blood with the remainder being recycled into my body.

I was taken to the apheresis room where I was briefed by two very competent nursing sisters. I would have to lie on my back almost motionless for about 4 hours whilst coupled to the machine. This high-tech machine was like a very sophisticated centrifuge which had a rotary head spinning at high speed which separated the blood into its various components according to their relative densities. The CD34$^+$ cells would be selectively removed and stored in strong plastic bags.

Blood would be drawn from an intravenous needle in my right arm, would pass through the machine and be returned to another intravenous needle in my left arm. Before the process could begin a suitable vein in my right arm had to be found. Once this was done, I was coupled up to the machine. They elected to use the existing drip in my left arm to return the blood.

As the machine whizzed away, a buff-coloured liquid (stem cells) was being separated out of my blood. I marvelled at the miracles of modern medicine. Not long into the process, the sister picked up problems with the return into my left arm and had to insert a needle into another vein. Soon thereafter, the vein they had chosen in my right arm began to collapse under suction and they had to find a better candidate. (Little did they realise that they were inadvertently contributing to my record daily tally of nine needles!)

Once all the hiccups were sorted out it was plain sailing and I dozed off whilst the lengthy process continued. I was awoken with the news that we were done and the sisters informed me that they had been able to bag enough stem cells for six transplants. In answer to prayer there truly had been an abundant harvest of stem cells – all glory to God!

Discharge Day

Since the mobilisation and harvesting was now complete, I was allowed a week's break before my stem cell transplant was to take place.

I wrote in my diary:

This is the day the LORD has made. We will rejoice and be glad in it. —Psalm 118:24 NLT

Before returning to Sabie I spent a little time with my sister Laura and niece Michelle who were visiting from the USA. It was great to connect with them and to catch up on all their news, but it ended with a rather tearful farewell which I hoped would not be the last.

Even though one has faith, there are certain times when one's emotions push through. Rather than burying them and continuing stoically, I believe we should acknowledge them as being part of the richness of life. After all, we are social and emotional beings!

Lessons Learnt

- We should realise that our faith is of greater worth than gold and that it will be refined and tested by fiery trials.

- God invites us to call on Him in times of trouble or crisis and promises to deliver us.

- We must have an understanding or revelation of both the power and the compassion of God.

- As we pray for healing (or for anything else for that matter), we should pray the Word of God and claim the promises of God rather than merely focusing on the problem.

- We should take medication in faith that it will be effective and accomplish what it is intended to do as quickly as possible.

- Realise that cancer is not for sissies. Overcome your fears by exercising faith. See yourself as an over-comer; the "Ultimate Survivor".

- We can be specific in our prayers and even pray for good blood results and effective treatment.

Key Facts

- Cancer patients undergoing chemotherapy often have reduced immunity and must be careful of infection.

CHAPTER 9

A LONG, LONELY BATTLE

No one enters an isolation ward for a stem cell transplant without a certain sense of trepidation. I had been forewarned by one of the sisters back in Nelspruit of its potential challenges. Far from wanting to instil fear in me, she just wanted me to be psychologically prepared for what lay ahead. So, just like a runner entering the renowned Comrades Ultra Marathon knows that it is going to require a huge amount of mental and physical endurance, I knew that things could be challenging, but I'd decided I was in it for the long haul so I had better make the best of it.

Some of the rooms in ward 20 overlooked a golf estate which was also a nature reserve, so I had prayed for a "room with a view" hoping that having a view of nature would help to lift my spirits during my times alone. I was not disappointed. My diary has the entry: *"Checked into Room 11 in Ward 20 – a room with a view. Thank you, Lord – You answer prayer!*

Desi helped me unpack all my goods and settle in. I had brought along plenty of things to keep me busy should I need them: my Bible, guitar, laptop, magazines, Christian books, binoculars etc. but I was also looking forward to a bit of solitude. Little did I realize that in many ways I would be kept quite busy during the coming weeks. I also had my own kettle, long-life milk, coffee, tea, sour sweets and snacks to remind me that I was loved.

On my admission there was the usual battery of blood and microbiological tests. Then, as a matter of course, they found a vein and put up a drip to hydrate me in preparation for chemo. My vitals were also checked (blood pressure, pulse, temperature and oxygen saturation). This was to happen every two hours, day and night for the rest of my stay. It disrupted my sleep patterns at first, but after a few nights I was almost oblivious of it happening and went straight back to sleep. More challenging was the phlebotomist coming in at 4am every morning to draw blood.

High Dose Chemo

The next day (designated Day minus three) I was treated to my first dose of Melphalan in what is known as "high-dose chemotherapy." When they say high dose, they mean it! I received something like ten times the dosage that would normally be administered in other treatments. The idea was for the Melphalan to all but kill off my bone marrow so that it could later be regenerated using my stem cells. It's a pretty drastic measure, something like death and resurrection. If your bone marrow fails to regenerate, you're pretty much done for. So, I deliberately and prayerfully put my life in the hands of the One called "the Resurrection and the Life".

The high dosage would also increase side-effects like nausea, so I was pre-dosed with an anti-nausea infusion and I had to suck ice to try to prevent the developmentof sores in my mouth and throat. The Melphalan dose was then run in rapidly. The next day I had a repeat dosage of the drug. My diary that day reads as follows:

Melphalan drip in my arm started burning and arm began swelling, so senior sisters came and quickly moved drip to my right arm. The rest of the chemo went okay. Felt nauseous at supper but ate my food anyway. Thankfully in all my treatments I have never thrown up. PTL! (Praise the Lord)

For the next several days I was fairly tired and weak and I struggled with nausea. I was determined to keep on eating solid foods for the duration of my isolation if at all possible. Many patients can't face the thought of food so go over to intravenous feeding. This can present challenges with one's drip and in any case one has to revert to solid food before one can be discharged.

Saying grace and blessing the food before meals took on a new meaning and significance. We had friends who were lifelong missionaries in Africa and they had had to eat the strangest things during their travels. They tried to eat everything set before them in order to show respect to their hosts and not to cause offence. They had taught us the missionary's prayer of grace which is simply: "Lord, I'll put it down if you'll keep it down." I'll admit, I prayed this prayer several times during isolation. It was not that the food was poor; it was just that my mouth and throat were dry and even the smell of food made me nauseous.

I found that I had no craving for sweet biscuits or chocolates and I had little sense of taste. I much preferred savoury snacks and plain salted Lays Chips became my staple diet between meals. (Desi jokes about our owning shares in the company). A dietician advised me on what I, as an immune-compromised patient, could and couldn't eat and she also recommended sour sweets as an alternative to regular sweets since sweet things tend to enhance nausea. This was good advice and I ended up guzzling sour worms and sour jelly beans.

Born Again

The day of my stem cell infusion, or "Day Zero" as it is referred to, arrived. The medical staff made a real fuss of this landmark event, likening it to a rebirth. My diary records this prayer that I prayed:

Day of rebirth! We are born again by the incorruptible seed of the Word of God. May my bone marrow be born again by incorruptible seed from my stem cell infusion!

They took photos of Desi holding the bag of my stem cells before they connected it to my drip and quickly ran in the buff- coloured liquid on which my very life depended. The whole process took only twenty minutes and seemed like a bit of an anti-climax.

To make sure that I was stable and healthy, I was hooked up to a monitor which kept a continuous record of my vitals for the next eighteen hours. It would periodically squeeze my arm in order to take my blood pressure. Despite some discomfort I had a reasonable night's rest.

Life in Isolation

I looked forward to Desi's daily visits and to visits by my son Stephen and eldest daughter Gina who both lived in Pretoria. They were a source of strength and encouragement to me. They looked rather strange decked out in their masks, gloves, aprons and hair nets. My youngest, Nicole, called me periodically from London. I was also aware of solid prayer support from the church back in Sabie and from my colleagues in ministry.

My daily Bible readings were a lifeline to me and I recorded in my diary some of the key Scriptures that spoke to me. When I was able, I would take up my guitar and sing worship songs. Singing was difficult because my mouth and throat were dry and sore from the chemo. Despite my croaky voice, the nurses loved this and would sometimes congregate in the ante-room and listen.

A Long, Lonely Battle

I tried to stay fit by doing some daily exercise. To this end I'd brought along a step, but found that step exercises were a bit too strenuous for me in my weakened state. As a result, I resorted to vigorous walking on the spot and several stretching exercises. (The step came in handy for one of my nurses who was short in stature and struggled to reach some of the instruments above my bed).

I would also keep an eye on the neighbouring golf estate for signs of wildlife. A group of Blesbok were frequent visitors and I would take up my binoculars to have a good look at them. There was also some birdlife around a near-by dam to keep me from getting bored.

The term 'isolation' is a bit of a misnomer since my nurses were often in and out to attend to my drip, bring in my food, give me my medication etc. The cleaners also followed a rigorous daily cleaning and sterilising regimen. My overseeing doctor would also do his daily rounds to check up on his patients. He was clear and thorough in explaining the process I was going through and also very encouraging. About halfway through my confinement he said that I was "cruising through the process." On another day he said that I had the highest haemoglobin result in the whole of Ward 20 (Ward 20 has some 30 rooms.) This was something to be thankful for.

Infection

Because white blood cells and platelets have a short lifespan their counts drop the most rapidly after high-dose chemotherapy, whilst red blood cells can survive for up to 115 days. As was expected, my white blood cell counts dropped to zero in a few days, and my platelet counts also plummeted. In this condition one has very little immunity and infections are fairly common.

Fortunately, I did not develop mucositis which occurs when cancer treatments break down the rapidly dividing epithelial cells lining the gastro-intestinal tract. This leaves the mucosal tissue open to infection and ulceration. This is apparently fairly difficult to treat. However, on day seven after my transplant, I developed a systemic infection and my temperature started to rise. I was put on antibiotics and blood was drawn in order to isolate and identify the offending organism. It turned out to be a bacterium that is normally found in the gut. (Klebsiella pneumoniae.) Because my resistance was so low it had somehow managed to get through my intestinal mucosa and into my bloodstream and began to propagate as an opportunistic pathogen.

That morning I had read a Scripture referring to Jesus which had bearing on my circumstances. I also recorded my prayer:

> *Although he was a son, he learned obedience from what he suffered... (Hebrews 5:8). I prayed: "Lord, may I learn obedience through the things I am suffering. May my life and my faith come forth pure like gold refined in the fire."*

I had a rough night. My temperature eventually climbed to 40^0 C and I again developed rigors. I had the nurses jumping as they tried to control my temperature. By the next morning it was back to normal and I was feeling okay; just a little washed out. Fortunately, it was not a highly resistant "hospital bug" causing the infection, but one which proved to be very sensitive to antibiotics and as a result the infection was cleared up in a few days.

Nose Dive

A bit later that morning I went to the bathroom to brush my teeth. I suddenly felt very faint, so I tried to head back to my bed. I woke up some time later lying on the floor in a pool of blood. I had fallen and bashed my nose on the hard floor and had a nosebleed which took a couple of nurses about five hours to bring under control. This was because my platelet count was very low making me prone to bleeding.

Eventually the nurses inserted a specialized plug in my nose which stopped the bleeding. It was only removed four days later. I was confined to my bed for several days and was not allowed to move around in my room or do anything without the assistance of a nurse. Later in the day I received an emergency transfusion of platelets to reduce the danger of further bleeding. This was repeated the next day when I also received a blood transfusion. I chuckled wryly to myself as I thought back on the events of the past day. How the mighty had fallen! From "cruising through the procedure" I ended up taking a nosedive and being imprisoned in my bed.

Taking a shower with a drip in my arm had always been a challenge, but now I had to be extra careful not to faint or fall during the process. Desi was an expert at helping me perform my daily ablutions. I felt like a dependent child once again and was so thankful to have her loving support all through my long struggle. Somehow it was a special time of a deeper bonding between us.

My Stem Cells Graft

On Day 10 there was the first encouraging sign that the stem cell transplant had begun to graft as my leucocyte count moved from zero to 0.05. From then on the count began to climb daily in small increments. There are several different classes of leucocytes, the most critical one in this case being the neutrophils. Once my neutrophil count reached 0.5 the transplant would be deemed to have graft-ed and I would be ready to be discharged as I would have regained a small measure of resistance to infection.

Going Against Goliath

My platelets were a bit slower in grafting and during my last week in isolation I received a further two infusions of platelets. On day fifteen I messaged some of my colleagues and asked for prayer for a breakthrough. In cricket idiom, the runs had been trickling in, but it was time for me to bat a 20+ over. I wanted God to be glorified. They prayed fervently and by the next day both my neutrophil and my platelet counts had almost doubled – all glory to God.

The entry in my diary reads as follows:

> *Praise the Lord!*
> *Neutrophils 2*   *(doubled overnight)*
> *Platelets 34*   *(nearly doubled o/n)*
> *Haemoglobin 9,6* *(going up)*

> *Thank you, Lord for answering the prayers of many. We hit some boundaries. I give you the glory! You can ask for anything in My name, and I will do it, so that the Son can bring glory to the Father. (14) Yes, ask Me for anything in My name, and I will do it!* —John 14:13-14 NLT

Based on these encouraging blood results I was discharged from Ward 20 on Day 16. I had been in isolation for 22 days. What a pleasure to have my drip removed and to be able to walk freely once again. What a joy to finally pack my bags and to bid the friendly staff goodbye. As we left the building I was overcome with emotion; I felt like a prisoner set free.

This Scripture encapsulates my emotions on that day:

> *But for you who fear My name, the Sun of Righteousness will rise with healing in His wings. And you will go free, leaping with joy like calves let out to pasture.* —Malachi 4:2 NLT

A Long, Lonely Battle

Key Facts

- One has to be mentally and spiritually prepared to endure the challenges of a stem cell transplant followed by recovery in an isolation ward.

- Your vital signs are monitored every two hours for the duration of your stay in isolation and blood samples are taken daily.

- High-dose chemotherapy administered before a stem cell transplant is intended to virtually kill off the bone marrow so that it can later be regenerated.

- High-dose chemotherapy is accompanied by considerable side effects like nausea, dry mouth, sore throat, loss of taste, weakness and diarrhoea.

- After high-dose chemotherapy one has almost no resistance for a period of time since one has no white blood cells. Platelet counts also plummet, whilst red blood cells survive a little longer.

- During the most critical period the patient invariably receives whole blood and platelet transfusions.

- A limited number of daily visitors are allowed and they have to wear protective clothing to prevent endangering the patient.

- Medical staff are on the lookout for signs of infection and are quick to act should this occur.

- Infused stem cells take a while to "graft", but eventually begin to repopulate the bone marrow which starts producing the different classes of blood cells.

- Dieticians will advise on which foods are permissible for an immune-compromised patient to eat. You may also wish to experiment with different snacks to suit your taste.

- *God is our refuge and strength, an ever-present help in trouble.* **(Psalm 46:1)**

Chapter 10

Bouncing Back

On my discharge from hospital we returned to our Benoni base for a few more days. I had to remain in the vicinity of the hospital until I had a final consultation with my haematologist. If he gave me the all-clear, we would be able to return to our home in Sabie.

When one has been through the fires of testing, one appreciates life's daily blessings so much more. I well remember how good my first home-cooked meal, lovingly prepared by my mother-in-law, tasted. Going for a daily walk with Desi around the grounds was another of life's privileges. I also recall relaxing in a chair on the sun porch and catching up with some friends via phone calls or WhatsApp. Life just seemed so much more valuable and relationships with people more important and precious!

We are taught in the Scriptures to number our days; in other words, to value them and make the best use of them. *Teach us to number our days aright, that we may gain a heart of wisdom.* (**Psalm 90:12**)

When one has had a stem cell transplant, one literally has to number one's days beginning at day zero which is the day of the transplant. It takes an average patient approximately 100 days to regain his or her strength and to get back to normal. During this period, one has to be very cautious about the fact that one may be immune-suppressed and take the necessary precautions of wearing a face mask in public and of social distancing in order to prevent picking up infectious diseases.

One's diet is also a priority. A large percentage of our white blood cells locate in the epithelial layers of our digestive tract. Their purpose is to form a barrier against potential infection. Certain foods, even some considered to be healthy, must be avoided since they contain live bacteria or yeasts. I was instructed to avoid yoghurt, non-irradiated nuts, honey, salt and pepper, undercooked meat or poultry, etc. Even the use of probiotics was considered dangerous as long as my immunity was low. I was also advised to avoid restaurants and fast-food outlets or any situation where food might have been re-heated completely.

Because of the impact of high-dose chemotherapy, the digestive tract's ability to digest protein is impaired for some time, so I was encouraged by the hospital dietician to continue using my hydrolysed whey-protein sports supplement in order to gain weight and strength. She also prescribed a vitamin-rich, nutritious shake between meals.

On Day 19 I had a consultation with my haematologist. My blood tests were good and he was pleased with my progress. He wrote out a prescription for several prophylactic drugs and gave me the green light to return to my home in Sabie.

Homecoming

The next day Desi drove us back to our home in the beautiful town of Sabie. There was a welcoming party of four church members to greet us on our arrival. They helped us offload our heavily laden car and quickly took their leave, somewhat fearful of compromising my health. I wrote in my diary that day:

Thank you, Lord for our safe arrival! Thank you, Lord that You kept our home and possessions safe! It's great to be home. Hallelujah!!!

Bouncing Back

I was quickly back in the saddle when it came to my pastoral responsibilities. I immediately took care of some administrative issues and then on Day 30 I preached again for the first time. It went well; it was great to be back in action fulfilling my calling. I took the necessary precaution of wearing a face mask and one of my church leaders requested the congregation to keep their distance from me. However, we are a charismatic church and members are used to greeting one another with a warm hug. Therefore, before I could take any defensive action I was enthusiastically hugged by a couple of the older ladies in the congregation as they greeted me after the service!

During my transplant I had lost 8 kg of weight and nearly all my hair, and I looked pale and gaunt. Over the next few weeks I exercised regularly and ate well and gradually began to regain my strength and weight. By Day 33 I was walking 5 km and exercising my arms using dumbbells. I gradually increased the pace and intensity of my exercise program. I soon took to the hills on my mountain bike and was surprised to find that I broke some of my personal best segment times as recorded on the Strava App on my smart phone. It seemed that I had more energy and strength than before my transplant.

On Day 41 we drove through to Witbank for a consultation with my haematologist. He already had the results of my blood tests taken a few days earlier. Everything looked good! My white blood cell counts were back in the normal range and my M-protein cancer marker was at zero. He said the stem cell transplant had been a great success. We discussed a future maintenance chemotherapy regimen and then he dismissed us with the good news that I could return to my normal lifestyle since my immunity was back to normal. It was yet another miracle that I was back to normal within 40 days rather than the usual 100 days.

Surely, the same Spirit that raised Christ from the dead was at work in my mortal body!

> *If the Spirit of him who raised Jesus from the dead is living in you, he who raised Christ from the dead will also give life to your mortal bodies through his Spirit, who lives in you.* —Romans 8:11

True Zero

At ACT Clinic it is normal protocol to take a bone marrow biopsy and aspiration from MM patients 100 days after a stem cell transplant. 100 days for me coincided with our church network's annual conference in Pretoria so I arranged to have the biopsy taken before the TCN conference. Desi and I would then attend the conference and by the time it was over the biopsy results would hopefully be available. This would mean we could have an important final consultation with my haematologist. Fortunately, this second bone marrow biopsy was quickly and efficiently performed. Although quite painful, it was nothing like the horrific ordeal I had endured during my diagnosis about ten months prior.

Well, after an inspiring conference and a few days' holiday at a country resort, the day of the consultation arrived with us both feeling strangely confident and peaceful. My haematologist informed us that my biopsy results were particularly good. In fact, they were the best post-transplant results the ACT Clinic had ever recorded for an MM patient. The clinic had existed for some ten years but in that time they had somehow never recorded what is known as a "true zero" result from a biopsy until mine came along. The tests showed that there were less than one in a million abnormal plasma cells in my bone marrow (in other words zero abnormal cells). The test had been repeated several times, each time with the same result; it was their first "true zero." This was a cause for some celebration at the unit and for us as well. We shared the good news with our family and friends celebrating the fact that, "God is good all the time, and all the time God is good".

Maintenance Chemotherapy

MM patients in remission are commonly put on what is termed as "maintenance chemotherapy" as a safeguard against any remaining cancer cells making a comeback. I was required to inject myself weekly with Valtib (borte-zomib) for three weeks in a row after which I would enjoy a week's respite. I also took the drug prednisone (a steroid) simultaneously.

The Valtib had virtually no side effects other than caus-ing red welts at the site of the injections. Fortunately, these were on my belly which was generally concealed except when I went swimming. The steroids again caused wake-fulness resulting in the need for me to take a sleeping tab-let on the first night after I took the meds.

Once every twelve weeks I would have blood tests prior to consulting with my oncologist. She would monitor my blood results to confirm that all was well and that I was still in remission. Whilst I was at her rooms I would also have an infusion of a bisphosphonate (zoledronic acid) to strengthen and restore my bones. Zoledronic acid scav-enges calcium from the blood and deposits it in the skele-ton. Apparently, bones which were perforated and weak-ened by the activity of MM can restore in time. Periodic bisphosphonate infusions aid the process.

Miraculously, life returned to normality for me. I was fit and well and regained my strength and all the weight I had lost. In fact, in some respects I was stronger than before my diagnosis. My blood counts confirmed that all was well; even my hair grew again! Thankfully, I was able to resume all my pastoral duties and fulfil my calling. This blissful state of affairs prevailed for eleven months…

Lessons Learnt

- Fiery tests help us appreciate life's daily blessings so much more.

Key Facts

- Taking precautions against infections and being careful about one's diet are important considerations for an immune-suppressed post-transplant patient.

- The success of a stem cell transplant is assessed by performing a bone marrow biopsy and aspiration in addition to the regular blood tests.

- Prophylactic antibacterial and antiviral drugs are often prescribed for post-transplant patients.

- MM patients in remission are commonly put on maintenance chemotherapy as a safeguard against any remaining cancer cells making a comeback.

- Periodic bisphosphonate infusions aid the process of the restoration of weakened and perforated bones.

CHAPTER 11

FIGHTING THE GOOD FIGHT

As the Apostle Paul approached the end of his earthly life he was able to say these words: *"I have fought the good fight, I have finished the race, I have kept the faith."* **(2 Timothy 4:7).** The question I have to ask myself is, will I be able to say the same?

You're probably reading this book because you have been diagnosed with cancer or know someone fighting this dread disease. From the preceding chapters it is clear that cancer is as much a spiritual battle as it is a physical one. I believe I have been through a few courses in the school of faith and I believe it could be helpful to share with you what I have learnt.

The Importance of Faith

> *...without faith it is impossible to please God, because anyone who comes to him must believe that he exists and that he rewards those who earnestly seek him.* —Hebrews 11:6

Faith is important to God; it pleases Him. We see here that there are two key things that we must believe about God: that He exists and that He rewards those who seek Him with all of their hearts. There are great rewards in pursuing God!

The importance of faith is underlined by the fact that Jesus was always on the lookout for faith and celebrated it whenever He found it. We have the example of the Centurion who sought healing for his servant who was desperately ill. Jesus was willing to go to his home, but the centurion replied, *"Lord, I do not deserve to have you come under my roof. But just say the word, and my servant will be healed.* **(Matthew 8:8)** *When Jesus heard this, he was astonished and said to those following him, "I tell you the truth, I have not found anyone in Israel with such great faith.* **(Matthew 8:10)**

Then there was the Canaanite Woman who sought deliverance for her demonized daughter – Jesus seemed to be terribly rude to her, but she persisted. Finally, he said, *"Woman, you have great faith! Your request is granted."* **(Matthew 15:28)**. Jesus will still be looking for faith when He returns. He asks the question: *"...when the Son of Man comes, will he find faith on the earth?"* **(Luke 18:8)**

When you travel to a foreign country you need to exchange your local currency into that of the foreign country in order to be able to trade. I call faith "the currency of the Kingdom." We need it to be able to do business in the Kingdom of God, to be able to trade. It's the means by which we're saved, by which our prayers are answered, healing is appropriated and demonic powers are defeated. This is confirmed by the following two Scriptures:

> **Therefore I tell you, whatever you ask for in prayer, believe that you have received it, and it will be yours.** —Mark 11:24

> **If any of you lacks wisdom, he should ask God, who gives generously to all without finding fault, and it will be given to him. But when he asks, he must believe and not doubt, because he who doubts is like a wave of the sea, blown and tossed by the wind. That man should not think he will receive anything from the Lord; he is a double-minded man, unstable in all he does.** —James 1:5-8

The message is clear: if we have faith in God our prayers will be answered. However, if we doubt, we should not think we will receive anything from the Lord.

I have two similar sayings which sum up the importance of faith:

"Great faith honours God and God honours great faith"

"God puts no limits on faith and faith puts no limits on God." *For nothing is impossible with God. (Luke 1:37).* Let's not limit God to the dimensions of our finite minds!

Defining Faith

Faith is not a mystical, ethereal thing. When you face a challenge people often say, "Just have faith," but to me that is an incomplete sentence. Faith needs to have a focus; faith needs to have an object. True faith is centred on the character of God and the Word of God. One should rather say, "Have faith in God" or "Have faith in the promises of God." This is indeed what Jesus said when his disciples marvelled at the fig tree He had cursed:

Have faith in God," Jesus answered. —Mark 11:22

There is a key verse in the Bible which we could say defines faith: *Now faith is the substance of things hoped for, the evidence of things not seen.* —Hebrews 11:1 NKJV

The Greek word translated "substance" here is *"hupostasis." "Hupo"* means under and *"stasis" means* to stand. So, faith is literally "that which stands under." It is a substance, something solid, like the foundation of a building which stands under and supports the superstructure. If we have faith, we will stand like a house built on a rock and not be shaken.

Faith is also *"the evidence of things not seen"* – faith relates to the invisible realm. We exercise faith when the answer to our prayers is not yet seen. When it does materialise or become seen, faith has done its work and is no longer really needed. As believers, *"We live by faith, not by sight..."* **(2 Corinthians 5:7).** We should not merely operate by our five natural senses but should see through the eye of faith and sense things in the spiritual realm even before they manifest in the physical realm.

Hope is also mentioned; it seems to precede faith. I like to refer to hope as the raw material and to faith as the catalyst which goes to work on that raw material, hope, in order to turn what we believe for into a reality.

We need to have a hope, a dream or a vision otherwise there is no feedstock for our faith. Then our faith needs to go to work on that hope in order to materialise it. Faith will turn your hopes into realities; the invisible into the visible; the ethereal into the material.

What Faith Is Not

I believe we can get a clearer picture of what faith is by pointing out what it is not.

There is a clear distinction between faith and presumption:

A presumptuous person decides what he or she wants and tries to twist God's arm to get it. Oftentimes there is a selfish motive. *When you ask, you do not receive, because you ask with wrong motives, that you may spend what you get on your pleasures.* **(James 4:3)**

The devil tried to get Jesus to jump from the temple and presume on God's protection, but Jesus would not put God to the test. There is a world of difference between faith and presumption.

Faith is not merely positive thinking:

There is natural power in positive thinking. Some unbelievers are able to give up smoking by sheer will power. But there is supernatural power in faith based on God and His Word. New agers think positive, believers think promises.

Faith is not a denial of the facts:

Denial is often based on fear, not in faith. People are too afraid to face the problem so, like the proverbial ostrich with its head in the sand, they pretend the threat doesn't exist. Unfortunately, many people diagnosed with cancer are living in denial to their own detriment. Denial is running from the facts.

Faith Faces Facts

> *Without weakening in his faith, he [Abraham] faced the fact that his body was as good as dead—since he was about a hundred years old—and that Sarah's womb was also dead.* —Romans 4:19

Abraham, the archetype of faith, faced the facts about his age and physical limitations. I encourage you to face the facts about your situation in faith. Face the facts about your medical condition.

Without weakening in my faith I had to face the fact that I had a disease called Multiple Myeloma which was wreaking havoc in my body. However, at the same time, I had to be convinced too of the truth of God's Word which says; *"...by his [Jesus'] wounds you have been healed."* **(1 Peter 2:24)**

Sometimes we have to exercise faith over a period of time before it is rewarded. Abraham had to wait something like seventeen years before Isaac, the child of promise, was born. During the waiting our faith must grow stronger, not weaker. Like Abraham we must become fully persuaded that God has the power to do what He has promised.

> *Yet he did not waver through unbelief regarding the promise of God, but was strengthened in his faith and gave glory to God, being fully persuaded that God had power to do what he had promised.* —Romans 4:20-21

The Power of the Spoken Word

> *By faith we understand that the worlds were framed by the word of God, so that the things which are seen were not made of things which are visible.* —Hebrews 11:3 NKJV

I believe in a creation which was 'ex-nihilo' – out of nothing – God spoke the elements (atoms) into being and then spoke the visible creation into being. The elements are the invisible building blocks of all that we can see. In this way God framed the world by His Word. So, we see that there was incredible power in the spoken words of God. Therefore, remembering that we are made in the image of God, we must realise that our words also carry weight. In a sense we frame our own worlds by the words we speak over ourselves, either negative or positive.

> *Death and life are in the power of the tongue, and those who love it will eat its fruit.* —Proverbs 18:21 NKJV. *Words kill, words give life; they're either poison or fruit—you choose.* —Proverbs 18:21 MSG

If even our natural words have influence, how much more weight and power do our words carry when we speak the very Word of God?

When God called Jeremiah, He touched his mouth and said:

> ***Now, I have put my words in your mouth...*** **Then, He went on and said,** ***...I am watching to see that my word is fulfilled.*** —Jeremiah 1:9,12

If God gives you a word, (e.g. a Scripture which becomes a personal Word or rhema to you, or a prophetic word) speak it out over your life and release its power. Your body, your soul, your circumstances, even the devil needs to hear it!

Faith needs a vehicle of expression. One of the ways faith is expressed is through words.

Faith Speaks

> *"The word is near you; it is in your mouth and in your heart," that is, the word of faith we are proclaiming: That if you confess with your mouth, "Jesus is Lord," and believe in your heart that God raised him from the dead, you will be saved.*
> —Romans 10:8-9

Here we are reading about the "word of faith" as it relates to salvation. By confessing our faith we're saved. Faith needs to be in two places: in your heart and in your mouth. The word of faith must be spoken out. Unfortunately, unbelief also speaks. Jesus said that *the mouth speaks what the heart is full of* **(Matthew 12:34)** – the two work in synergy. If my heart is full of unbelief, I will not speak faith; I'll speak fear and negativity. In the same way, if my heart is full of hate, I will not speak words of love. But if my heart is full of faith I will speak words of faith.

Let us pray that our words will be pure and powerful:

May the words of my mouth and the meditation of my heart be pleasing in your sight, O LORD, my Rock and my Redeemer. —Psalm 19:14

Let us pray for instructed tongues to bless others:

The Sovereign LORD has given me an instructed tongue, to know the word that sustains the weary. —Isaiah 50:4

The Spoken Word and Healing

Now, let's take a practical and look at the spoken word and healing. The Centurion whose servant was ill knew the authority and power in Jesus' words. He said, *"Lord, I do not deserve to have you come under my roof. But just say the word, and my servant will be healed."* **(Matthew 8:8).** Jesus didn't pray a prayer for people to be healed, He just said a word: *"Be clean!"* **(Mark 1:41)** *"Get up! Pick up your mat and walk."* **(John 5:8)** *"Stretch out your hand."* **(Matthew 12:13)** *"Lazarus, come out!"* **(John 11:43)**

The question many of us ask is, "Can we do the same?" The answer is yes. We see the disciples doing the same thing at the gate beautiful: *Then Peter said, "Silver or gold I do not have, but what I have I give you. In the name of Jesus Christ of Nazareth, walk."* **(Acts 3:6)**

In Lystra... *Paul... saw that he [a lame man] had faith to be healed and called out, "Stand up on your feet!" At that, the man jumped up and began to walk.* **(Acts 14:9-10)**

The Prayer of Faith

Based on what I've just said above, some say we should never pray for healing, only command it, but I think that's taking it a bit too far! There is evidence in the Scripture of people praying for healing. However, when we pray we must pray the "Prayer of Faith."

> *Is any one of you sick? He should call the elders of the church to pray over him and anoint him with oil in the name of the Lord. And the prayer offered in faith will make the sick person well; the Lord will raise him up.* —James 5:14-15

When it comes to healing we can pray in faith. (See my example of a prayer for healing based on the promises of Scripture, on page 74). Healing is the revealed will of God. His Word is His will and His will is His Word. There are many promises of healing in God's Word. So, in this instance I don't believe we should pray, "If it be Thy will," since we are sure that God's will is to heal. I can also say this with confidence because God actually introduced Himself to us as Jehovah Rophe, the LORD our healer saying, *I am the LORD, who heals you.* **(Exodus 15:26)**

("Jehovah or Yahweh" is translated from the Hebrew YHWH as LORD and *"rophe"* means healer.) God was saying in effect, "healing is who I am."

One of the reasons Jesus came was to reveal the Father to us. In this regard, Jesus demonstrated that it is the will of God to heal by healing the sick wherever He went. There are some interesting verses in the Gospels which summarise the very comprehensive healing ministry of Jesus; here is but one:

> *Jesus went throughout Galilee, teaching in their synagogues, preaching the good news of the king-dom, and healing every disease and sickness among the people. News about him spread all over Syria, and people brought to him all who were ill with various diseases, those suffering severe pain, the demon-possessed, those having seizures, and*

the paralyzed, and he healed them. —Matthew 4:23-24

Faith Expressed by Obedient Action

We've seen that faith is expressed through words but now let's look at how faith can be expressed through our actions. The account of the paralysed man lowered through the roof by his friends is well known. How Jesus perceived their actions is interesting:

> **When Jesus saw their faith, he said to the paralytic, "Son, your sins are forgiven."** —Mark 2:5

I'd like you to consider whether or not your faith works. Is it true faith that takes action and gets results? Can someone see your faith by your actions?

Many of the miracles of Jesus demanded action:

In the miracle of the turning of water to wine at the wedding in Cana of Galilee people expressed their faith by their obedient action: *His mother [Mary] said to the servants, "Do whatever he [Jesus] tells you."* **(John 2:5)** The servants obeyed and a miracle resulted.

In the miracle of the healing of lame man at the pool of Bethesda, Jesus gave a simple, but challenging command: *"Get up! Pick up your mat and walk."* **(John 5:8).** The man obeyed and walked after many years being a cripple.

In the miracle of the healing of the man born blind, Jesus again gave instructions which required action on the part of the blind man.*"Go,"* he told him, *"wash in the Pool of Siloam." So the man went and washed, and came home seeing.* **(John 9:7)**

Faith doesn't sit on the fence in indecision; faith acts decisively. We see how a bold, decisive Peter got out of the boat and walked on the water in response to Jesus' invitation, "Come!" **(Matthew 14:29)**. I encourage you to rather be a wet water walker than a dry boat sitter.

Faith doesn't just pray; it also knows when to obey. When the children of Israel were hemmed in between the Egyptian army and the Red Sea, Moses cried out to the Lord in prayer:

> ***Then the LORD said to Moses, "Why are you crying out to me? Tell the Israelites to move on. Raise your staff and stretch out your hand over the sea to divide the water so that the Israelites can go through the sea on dry ground..."*** —Exodus 14:15-16

Increasing Your Faith

I have a saying: "Impression without expression leads to depression." It would be wrong for me to merely "impress" you with this chapter on faith, so I would like to conclude it by giving you, my reader friend, two practical exercises which I believe will increase your faith for healing should you do them.

We read in Scripture how faith is imparted to us as we hear God's Word. *So then faith comes by hearing, and hearing by the word of God.* **(Romans 10:17 NKJV).** The more we hear God's Word and God's promises, the more our faith will grow.

I believe that the more so-called "gates" to our minds and hearts we use, the better. As we read God's written Word we are using the eye gate – we "see" it. As we say it out loud we are using the ear gate – we "hear" it. We can also picture or visualise the Scripture we are reading in a way that helps it come alive to us. This is another way of "seeing" God's Word. I believe we should also internalise God's Word by memorising portions that are especially relevant to us.

Exercise One

Why don't you read the following Scripture several times over?

> *Praise the LORD, O my soul, and forget not all his benefits— who forgives all your sins and heals all your diseases, who redeems your life from the pit and crowns you with love and compassion...* — Psalm 103:2-4

(It may be better for you to find it and read it from your own Bible).

Concentrate on seeing the words. Focus on the phrases "forgives all your sins" and "heals all your diseases".

Then speak to your soul as you say the Scripture out loud several times. Concentrate on hearing the words.

Then visualise the Lord's lifting you out of a deep muddy pit, His washing you off and forgiving you, His anointing and healing you and then His crowning you with His love and compassion.

Finally try to memorise the Scripture so that you can mutter it to yourself or meditate on it all day long.

Exercise Two

We increase our level of fitness and strength through exercise:

> *The apostles said to the Lord, "Increase our faith!" He replied, "If you have faith as small as a mustard seed, you can say to this mulberry tree, 'Be*

uprooted and planted in the sea,' and it will obey you. —Luke 17:5-6

At first glance it doesn't appear that Jesus responded to their request, but on a closer look we see He was encouraging them to exercise their faith in order to increase it. Faith speaks. They were to speak out authoritative words of command.

In South Africa, mulberry trees have been classified as undesirable invaders which should be eradicated. The cancer in your body is an undesirable invader as well. Address any cancer remaining in your body as an undesirable invader and command it to be uprooted and planted in the sea. Then speak life and health into your body. Do this daily for a week. There is life and death in the power of the tongue.

CHAPTER 12

DOWN FOR THE COUNT

When the young lad David killed the Philistine giant Goliath, the armies of Israel were greatly encouraged, rallied their ranks, and took on the Philistine army. They experienced a decisive victory that day. Unfortunately, that was not the end of David's problem with the Philistines. Years later when he was anointed as king, the Philistine army gathered again to challenge his kingship. And again, during his reign, David fought several more battles against his arch enemies, each time triumphing through God's guidance and help.

Unfortunately fighting cancer is something like fighting the Philistines; it is not a once-off battle, but a lengthy war of attrition. We might rejoice in winning a decisive battle only to discover sometime later that our enemy has rallied and reappeared to take us on yet again.

My successful stem cell transplant appeared to have been a decisive victory over multiple myeloma and I enjoyed eleven months of perfect health. Unfortunately, I was rudely awakened from my blissful, dreamlike existence by a bad blood result. My M-protein count had jumped from zero to seven indicating that something was clearly amiss. My oncologist expressed her disappointment saying wistfully, "It could have held off a bit longer," but to be sure she was correct in her assessment, arranged that I had a bone marrow biopsy to confirm if there was a resurgence of the cancer.

The biopsy confirmed the bad news that the cancer was back; in fact, my haematologist was quite alarmed that he could see a large percentage of abnormal plasma cells under the microscope. He was concerned about how rapidly I had relapsed and said that we would need to take decisive action to prevent the myeloma spreading further. The cancer had become resistant to bortezomib (my maintenance chemo drug) which was now as good as useless, so we discussed various other treatment options. He settled on a seven-drug cocktail abbreviated KRd–PACE. He decided to throw everything, including the kitchen sink at this recurring intruder!!

This was of course a huge disappointment to me and it all but floored me. All my expectations were dashed to the ground and I had to pick myself up emotionally and spiritually. My expectations were based on the information that, after a successful autologous stem cell transplant, the average expected disease-free timeframe is three years. Given the apparent success of my transplant, I had expected even more than that; perhaps seven years. However, I had only enjoyed a paltry eleven months of disease-free living before the battle lines were again drawn.

We called together our church leadership group to inform them of the latest disappointing developments. They encouraged Desi and me, and prayed with us. During the time of prayer, Jackie, a lady leader and close friend of ours, had a vision of Desi and me climbing a high mountain. When the going got particularly steep and difficult for us, somehow, supernaturally, a handrail appeared which steadied us and helped us. She felt it was God promising to be with us and help us, especially through the times of greatest difficulty. We held onto this word of encouragement through the next trying season.

The need for urgent action was underlined by another blood result. In a mere three weeks, my M-protein score had risen further, from seven to nineteen. I would be able to receive this radical chemotherapy only whilst under hospitalisation, so plans were quickly put in place for me to return to Netcare Pretoria East Hospital for the infusions. I was duly checked in to the hospital ward and my therapy began. It was a long, drawn out process with the various drugs slowly run into my system over a period of four days. Along with it there were the usual battles with intravenous needles and drips.

Two of the drugs (Kyprolis and Revlimid) were more recently developed and have fewer side-effects, whilst the rest were more classical chemotherapy drugs which arrest cell replication and have profound side-effects. Nausea, diarrhoea, mucositis and hair loss were to be expected. Fortunately, my prayers were again answered and I got off lightly. I did end up bald for a season, which in any event was quite fashionable, or so my younger parishioners assured me.

With the therapy successfully administered, I was discharged. Since I was immune-suppressed with my white cell count still very low, I spent the next few days in the vicinity of the hospital before getting the green light to return to Sabie.

The Valley of the Shadow of Death

I'd only been home for a couple of days when I began running a temperature which soon turned into a raging fever. Desi and I fought the fever right through a Saturday night and then called my haematologist early on the Sunday morning. He advised me to report to the casualty ward at our local hospital. This soon developed into a nightmare of an experience – the details of which I won't go into here. It was three hours before the doctor on duty arrived. Fortunately, in the interim, my oncologist had made arrangements to have me transferred to Nelspruit Mediclinic.

Had I remained in the local hospital; I'm convinced I would have died that night.

On arrival in Nelspruit, I was rushed into an isolation ward and immediately put on a drip with powerful broad-spectrum antibiotics since I had developed a dangerous systemic infection. I miraculously made it through that first night. The next morning when my oncologist did her rounds of the ward, she expressed her great relief that I had made it, because in her experienced opinion, it had been touch-and-go. She said that one of the contributing factors to my survival was my physical fitness which ensured that my blood pressure stayed rock solid in the normal range right through that first night. I'm convinced that I was also carried through by the chorus of prayer that resounded for me in the courts of heaven. My faithful shepherd had not left my side. I was reminded of the verse in Psalm 23 which reads: *Even though I walk through the valley of the shadow of death, I will fear no evil, for you are with me; your rod and your staff, they comfort me.* **(Psalm 23:4)**

This was by no means the end of this particular battle. As my infection levels were high and my neutrophil count extremely low, I was still very definitely in the danger zone. Over the next week I was infused with a variety of broad-spectrum antibiotics and my infection index (CRP) gradually came down from 494 to 66, when I was finally discharged. The microbiology laboratory was unable to isolate or identify the offending microorganism in their blood cultures.

The Journey to Hell

Although the infection was brought under control and my physical condition stabilised after my week in hospital, my mental condition was impacted negatively. I apparently began to have episodes of strange, uncontrolled behaviour. Over the next week these increased in frequency and duration. My poor wife had great difficulty in coping with my abnormal behaviour.

Mental issues or not, my haematologist was anxious that the myeloma relapse be brought under control, so within a week I was scheduled for my second round of the KRd-PACE chemo cocktail back in Pretoria. I was required to check in to the hospital ward by 10:00, so we planned to leave early on that same morning. Packing what was needed and getting the car loaded proved to be a nightmare for Desi because I had a couple of early morning behavioural episodes during the process. We eventually took to the road over an hour later than planned, but still with a good safety margin of time for the journey.

During the journey, I had several more mental episodes or seizures. Each time, my dear Desi was forced to pull over to the side of the road and wait until I came to my senses again. On one occasion I even tried to open my door to get out the vehicle whilst we were travelling at 120 km per hour. She had to cross a lane of traffic and screech to a halt at the side of the highway and convince me to stay in the car.

Some of my antics were a little more amusing. At one point Desi mentioned that she was getting a bit warm in her thick winter clothing, so no trouble to me, I soaked her hair with water from my water bottle. She rode for some distance with me holding the dribbling water bottle over her head. Talk about loony tunes! The occupants of overtaking vehicles gawped at us in bewilderment. We eventually arrived at the hospital over an hour late. Instead of the journey taking the usual four hours, it had taken a full six hours. Desi still thinks of it as the "Journey to Hell".

Rounds Two and Three

Before the medical team were able to begin my chemotherapy, they had to bring my mental episodes under control and so a neurologist was consulted. He had a technician come and fit me with all the necessary wires and
probes for an EEG (Electro encephalograph). They hoped
to record my brain waves overnight over a fourteen-hour
period in order to pinpoint the problem. Unfortunately, I
soon had an episode in which I locked myself in the bathroom and began ripping the probes off my head. My son,
who was visiting me at the time eventually managed to
open the bathroom door, but by that time it was too late;
the damage was done.

From about four hours of data my neurologist felt he
had been able to garner enough information to hazard a
diagnosis. They had also managed to record the onset of
the episode. He believed that I was having seizures like
those of epilepsy and put me on what he deemed to be
appropriate drugs. (Epilezine, Dopaquel, Zopax and Thi-
amine). I was not convinced in my spirit that this diagnosis
was correct. The severity of the episodes began to decline,
but in spite of the drugs I was taking, I continued having
other mental symptoms. My sleep was disturbed and errat-
ic and I had the weirdest, scariest hallucinations. One night
I was convinced that some evil-minded men were about to
blow up the hospital. It was all so very clear; I could see
the group of men and where they had placed the explo-
sives, so I rushed down the passage to warn the night staff
to evacuate the building or we were all about to die. I
chuckle now at my state of mind, but at the time these hallucinations were no laughing matter.

The neurologist eventually brought a semblance of control to my behaviour by adjusting the dosages of the drugs
so the medical team were able to begin administering a
second round of the seven-drug chemotherapy cocktail
(KRd–PACE). Once the chemo had been administered

over several days, I spent some time recuperating at my mother-in-law's home in Benoni.

ACT Clinic had been very kind and had provided the Kyprolis pro-bono for the first two rounds of treatment. My medical aid was however, unwilling to pay for the drug since it had not yet been approved for use in South Africa, so it was up to me to try and source some further supplies. There was some stock available in the country, but it was frightfully expensive. So, whilst I was still confined to hospital, my son Stephen helped me to withdraw funds from some of my retirement investments and I eventually imported enough of the drug from Turkey, at a much lower price, for a further three rounds of treatment.

My medical aid was also unwilling to pay for Revlimid which is also extremely expensive. ACT Clinic again came to the party and provided three cycles of treatment with Revlimid free of charge. I am very thankful for these interventions by ACT Clinic on my behalf which may well have saved my life.

Before my import of Kyprolis arrived, my next cycle of treatment was due, so my haematologist opted for a six-drug cocktail of all the other available drugs (Rd–PACE). By this time the chemotherapy had hardened my once prominent veins and it had become increasingly difficult for the staff to put up an intravenous drip, so we decided that it was time for me to have surgery to insert a "central line" or "port". This actually made things so much easier and I wondered why we had not done it sooner.

These three rounds of rather hectic chemotherapy took their toll on me and this period of time is somewhat blurred in my memory. I was still struggling with insomnia and an overactive imagination and I was also rambling and long-winded in conversation. At times I began to stutter or could not speak at all. The good news was that the chemotherapy treatment was going to target and bringing the cancer under control. Thankfully, after the third cycle of treatment my M-protein score was down to three. (During my relapse it had peaked at nineteen). It was therefore agreed that, as we proceeded with my treatment, we would lose five of the drugs and continue with only the more targeted Kd component (Kyprolis and Dexamethasone). Kd would be administered at my oncologist's rooms in Nelspruit so it was possible for us to return home once more after about two months on the "frontline" of the battle.

Holding on to the Handrail

For Desi this was a particularly trying time and she had to guard her heart against getting into self-pity. Not only was she visiting me in hospital daily, but she was also keeping an eye on her aged mother who had had a fall and was suffering from severe back pain. During this time, she had to take her mom for doctor's consultations, X-rays and ultimately for an operation. Desi very definitely had to hang onto the handrail and to remember that God loved her with an unending, unfailing love in spite of the circumstances.

When we start asking questions like "Why Lord?" or "Why me?", we are but a short step from falling into the quagmire of self-pity. It is far more helpful for us to ask "How Lord? How do you wish me to react at this time Lord? How will you be helping me as I face this struggle Lord?" Trials and tribulations will either make us BITTER or BETTER. When God allows us to be tested it is with a positive result in mind. He wants us to turn TESTS into TESTIMONIES. He wants us to grow more Christ-like in character. The apostle Paul, who faced many trials and much persecution said the following: ...*we also rejoice in our sufferings, because we know that suffering produces perseverance; perseverance, character; and character, hope.* **(Romans 5:3-4)**

If we looked around, we could see evidences of God's helping hand even in our darkest times. We could see that He had always provided a handrail for us to hang onto. For example, family and friends came to visit me in hospital when I was at a low ebb and were a source of hope and encouragement. Also, a very clear evidence of God's hand of protection became evident whilst we were in Pretoria and our home stood empty in Sabie. My brother Howard and his wife Cecile wished to visit the Kruger National Park so we encouraged them to stay over in our home for a night on their way down. On the only night our home was occupied in a space of about two months, my solar inverter failed and caught fire. At about two in the morning Howard, who happens to be an electrical engineer, was wakened to the sound of loud pops and bangs and the smell of acrid smoke. He rushed downstairs to find my solar inverter had caught fire. He quickly found a fire extinguisher and put out the blaze, then isolated the solar system electrically. Had he not been present, my log home definitely would have caught fire and probably would have burnt to the ground leaving us without home or possessions. God knew what was about to happen and put a rescue plan in place. Hallelujah!

A blessing of the person who fears God and whom God corrects is this: *You will know that your tent is secure; you will take stock of your property and find nothing missing.* **(Job 5:24)**

Lessons Learnt

- Fighting cancer is most often not a once-off battle, but a lengthy war. Disappointing relapses can occur.

- When we face hardships, it is far more helpful for us to ask, "How Lord?" than it is for us to ask, "Why Lord?"

- When God allows us to be tested it is with a positive result in mind. He wants us to turn tests into testimonies. He wants us to grow more Christ-like in character.

Key Facts

- Sometimes chemotherapy can only be administered whilst the patient is hospitalised so that the drugs can be infused very slowly and the patient's vital signs can be monitored.

- Aerobic and anaerobic exercise benefits heart-lung fitness which can help maintain blood pressure in the normal range. A steady blood pressure can help a patient survive serious infections.

- Systemic infections can result in high fevers which in turn can lead to mental problems.

CHAPTER 13

A MENTAL BATTLE

We are tripartite beings made up of spirit, soul and body. These three components of our being do not function in isolation, but are interdependent. Physical illness of the body can impact on our psychological well-being. The opposite is also true and many physical illnesses are psychosomatic in origin. Cancer and the severe treatment it sometimes requires, not only impacts on our physical body, but can also affect us mentally and emotionally.

Since it may be of much help to you if you are fighting cancer, I would like to share with you some of the mental challenges I faced after my relapse. The radical chemotherapy treatment I underwent and the severe systemic infection which resulted in a high fever, combined to create a "perfect storm" which not only hammered me physically, but mentally as well. I pick up my account where I left off in the previous chapter…

Home Again

It was good to be home on familiar turf once again; however, I was still both physically weak and mentally challenged and returning to work immediately was out of the question. My treatment had to continue and the plan was for me to commute to Nelspruit for ongoing chemotherapy weekly.

On hearing about my mental state, my oncologist was a bit reluctant to use Kyprolis (carfilzomib) again, even though my imported consignment of this costly drug had since arrived in the country. Kyprolis had not yet been approved for use in South Africa by SAHPRA, (the South African Health Products Regulatory Authority – the South African equivalent of the FDA). However, my oncologist had been given special permission to use the drug and I had been required to sign an indemnity allowing her to do so. Although it was being used successfully in several other countries around the world, reports indicated that on rare occasions Kyprolis had apparently caused side effects impacting the brain; a condition described by the acronym PRES (Posterior Reversible Encephalopathy Syndrome). (Drugs.com 2020) There were grave concerns that I was suffering from this syndrome.

A definitive test would be for me to undergo an MRI scan which would indicate if my brain had been negatively affected by the drug. The MRI scan came back clear, but there was still the question as to why I had been mentally affected, so in order to get more insight I was referred to a psychiatric hospital called AKESO to be evaluated further.

Watching and Praying

Before beginning with the program at AKESO, the psychiatrist attending to me wanted to have a clear diagnosis. She was not convinced that I was having seizures akin to epilepsy and was not happy with some of the medication that had been prescribed. So, in order to cleanse my system and be able to get a clear diagnosis, I was taken off all medication for a period of two days. This resulted in my having fairly severe withdrawal symptoms which included insomnia. My mind was hyperactive and I didn't sleep a wink for the full forty-eight-hour period.

What do you do when you can't sleep at all? The lights were out during the night and I was not supposed to read, so I elected to pray. I was inspired by the account of Jesus praying to His Father all through the night on a number of occasions. For instance, He spent a night in prayer before choosing the twelve disciples *(see Luke 6:12)* and then also spent a night alone in prayer on a mountain after the miracle of the feeding of the five thousand *(see Matthew 14:23)*. Hadn't He also warned the sleepy disciples saying, *"Watch and pray so that you will not fall into temptation. The spirit is willing, but the body is weak."*? **(Matthew 26:41)**

Praying for hours on end for two nights in a row was both a challenging and rewarding experience. It is amazing how much ground you can cover in prayer when you pray non-stop for nine hours. I would light on a topic and pray until I ran out of words. Then I would switch over to praying in other tongues for some time until fresh inspiration and revelation filtered into my mind enabling me to continue praying in English. This kind of teamwork in prayer between myself and the Holy Spirit kept me going for hours. The apostle Paul seemed to pray in the same way. He makes the statement: *For if I pray in a tongue, my spirit prays, but my mind is unfruitful. So what shall I do? I will pray with my spirit, but I will also pray with my mind...* **(1 Corinthians 14:14-15)**

I prayed for my family members, the church, the patients in AKESO, our future, my health etc. etc. My prayers were deeper and more profound than at other times and were accompanied with much emotion. I felt that I was praying more from my heart than from my head. We should not be afraid of expressing emotions in prayer. Consider this description of Jesus' prayer life: *During the days of Jesus' life on earth, he offered up prayers and petitions with loud cries and tears to the one who could save him from death, and he was heard because of his reverent submission.* **(Hebrews 5:7)**

After my first drug free day a technician fitted me with the necessary wires and probes for an EEG. They then recorded my brain waves for a full day. I warned my psychiatrist that the results might appear a bit unusual because

I had not slept at all and had spent a large part of the night praying in the Spirit. Fortunately, she is a believer and understands spiritual things so what I said was not too foreign to her. The results of the EEG showed no evidence of any seizures and as a result she made some significant changes to my prescribed medication. She eventually diagnosed that I had a symptom complex called delirium. This explained my episodes of strange behaviour and the very graphic hallucinations that I was having. Once the correct diagnosis had been made and appropriate medication had been prescribed, my mental condition improved fairly rapidly. I ascribe my excellent progress to good professional medical intervention as well as to answered prayer.

This poor man called, and the LORD heard him; he saved him out of all his troubles. —Psalm 34:6

The Valley of Weeping

Despite making some good progress, I was still rather tearful and somewhat depressed. I believe that much of this emotion was brought on by the prospect of our impending retirement. We had ministered in Sabie for almost thirty-four years and during that time had pioneered and established Living Waters Christian Church. They had been fruitful and fulfilling years, but we had told our leadership that we felt it was time to move on and leave the church to our younger and more energetic associate pastor. In any event, I had reached the ripe old age of sixty-five, which was the accepted norm for retirement within our church network (TCN).

We hoped to relocate to Pretoria in due course to be near two of our children and our three grandchildren. Because we were separated from them by some distance, we had missed so much of our grandchildren's early childhood development. It was our intention to become more involved in their lives and to be part of their upbringing.

A Mental Battle

During my tenure in Sabie I had overseen and been physically involved in the building of three phases of our church facilities and had also built our double-storey log cabin which had been our family home for more than twenty years. We loved the town and its people and our roots in the community ran deep, so I guess I was struggling with leaving all this behind and to come to terms with the major changes which were in the pipeline for us. All precipitated what I believe was a process of mourning that I went through. We mourn when there is a sense of loss. There is healing in tears and I had to work through some deep emotions before I could embrace the major transition before me.

As I think about my mental and emotional struggles I am reminded of Psalm 84 which is about people making pilgrimage to meet with God in Jerusalem:

> **What joy for those whose strength comes from the LORD, who have set their minds on a pilgrimage to Jerusalem. When they walk through the Valley of Weeping, it will become a place of refreshing springs. The autumn rains will clothe it with blessings. They will continue to grow stronger, and each of them will appear before God in Jerusalem.**
> —Psalm 84:5-7 NLT

Sometimes we first have to pass through a time of sorrow or weeping before we can enter into our future joy. We must not merely endure the time of sorrow, but transform it into a place of springs. As I relied on the Lord's strength and gradually walked through my mental and emotional "Valley of Weeping" it did indeed become for me a place of refreshing springs. Part of the battle had to do with my sense of identity.

In my pastoral ministry I had dealt with Christian men facing retrenchment or the challenges of retirement and had always counselled them to embrace their primary identity as sons of God. Men in particular gain much of their sense of identity from what they do as an occupation. If they are retrenched or end up retiring, they often go through an identity crisis. At such a time they often need reminding that the most important thing about them is not what they do, but who they are: beloved sons of God. Now the shoe was on the other foot and I had to live by my own words of counsel to others. I had always been fairly goal centred and prided myself on being able to get a job done. I didn't realise how much of my sense of purpose and worth came from tackling projects and doing things. Now, I would have to deepen my own sense of identity in the Lord and find new direction and purpose as I waited on Him.

Dear reader, you and I do not have to perform in order to earn or win God's love and acceptance. We simply need to receive His forgiveness and fatherly embrace and to revel in our identity as children of God. It's not what we do that really matters, but who we are. *How great is the love the Father has lavished on us, that we should be called children of God! And that is what we are!* **(1John 3:1)**

Cancer can result in the need for huge adjustments in one's lifestyle and may even signal the end of one's productive career. Responding positively to these changes is both an emotional and a spiritual battle.

Tackling the Spirit of Heaviness

I had hardly ever suffered from depression in my entire life and had certainly never had to rely on medication, so it was a new enemy I had to face. To have to take a daily dose of an anti-depressant was an anathema to me, but it was prescribed for me for six months. As a result of my own experience I now have more compassion for those living in this form of darkness and oppression and for those who are dependent on anti-depressants.

Sometimes the cause of depression is a physical condition like biochemical or hormonal imbalances in the body. In my case, my psychiatrist found that I had hypothyroidism (an underactive thyroid gland). This was probably an underlying contributor to my tiredness, tearfulness and depression. We are not sure what compromised my thyroid gland; perhaps it was the high dose chemotherapy I had endured or the high fevers that I had experienced as I fought infections. Whatever the cause, in addition to the anti-depressant my psychiatrist also prescribed a hormone supplement called Euthyrox in order to bring the level of the hormone thyroxin in my blood into the normal range. Initially I was also placed on one or two other drugs including an anti-psychotic in order to bring my delirium under control, but I was gradually weaned off these over the next few months.

The various drugs definitely helped me get back to my normal self, but I'm convinced they were not the only contributors. I firmly believe that depression can also have a spiritual dimension; that it is in fact a form of spiritual oppression and needs to be fought with spiritual weapons as well. I have dealt with depression in some of my counselees over my years of pastoral ministry and have witnessed amazing, almost instantaneous breakthroughs in some people's lives in response to prayer and "spiritual warfare." (Spiritual warfare is when a Christ follower exercises his/her spiritual authority and comes against spiritual forces of evil causing oppression in his or her own or another person's life). The prophet Isaiah refers to a spirit of despair or heaviness and how the Messiah will bring victory over this spirit. Mourning, despair and heaviness sound like depression to me!

> *[The Messiah would come to] ...comfort all who mourn, and provide for those who grieve in Zion— to bestow on them a crown of beauty instead of ashes, the oil of gladness instead of mourning, and a garment of praise instead of a spirit of despair...*
> —Isaiah 61:2-3

Once we have come under the authority of God in prayer, we can turn our attention to the enemy we face and directly address the "spirit of heaviness" or the spirit responsible for depression, bind it, and command it to leave us in Jesus' name. We don't have time to do a comprehensive study on spiritual warfare here, but these Scriptures give some further background on the subject:

> *[Jesus' words to His disciples]: I have given you authority to trample on snakes and scorpions and to overcome all the power of the enemy; nothing will harm you. (Luke 10:19) And these signs will accompany those who believe: In my name they will drive out demons; they will speak in new tongues... —Mark 16:17*

> *Submit yourselves, then, to God. Resist the devil, and he will flee from you. —James 4:7*

With my experience, and the above scriptures in mind, I actively fought off the spirit of heaviness and depression. I took authority over it and banished it from my life. I also quoted and claimed the promise in Paul's words to his timid disciple Timothy.

> *For God has not given us a spirit of fear, but of power and of love and of a sound mind.*
> —2 Timothy 1:7 NKJV

A Mental Battle

I believed and confessed that I had a sound mind. I can testify that I again have a sound mind and that depression is a thing of the past. The only medication I am taking now is a single daily dose of the hormone euthyrox.

A Prayer for Deliverance from Depression

Heavenly Father I submit to your rule and authority over my life. Jesus, Son of the Most High, I confess you to be my Lord. Thank you that you have given me authority to overcome all of the power of the Evil One in your Name.

Now Satan and demonic powers of darkness, I address you in Jesus' name. I come against the spirit of heaviness and depression and command it to leave me right now, never to return. I put on the garment of praise instead of the spirit of heaviness. I uproot sadness and despair and declare that you have no more place in my life. Sorrow and mourning flee! The joy of the Lord is my strength. Now I come against the spirit of fear and confusion. In Jesus' name I command it to leave right now. God has not given me a spirit of fear, but a spirit of love and of power and of a sound mind. I proclaim that I have victory in Jesus' mighty name! Amen.

Dear reader, if you are from a Western background as I am, you are probably finding what I've been saying to be rather strange and a bit "spooky spiritual." We westerners have been brought up with a worldview which is materialistic and which denies the reality of the spiritual realm. This is merely our skewed perception based on our background. I've come to realise that the spiritual realm is a profound reality and that sometimes the battles we face are spiritual in nature. Sometimes we have to take stock of

131

what's happening to us and discern whether it is a form of spiritual attack or oppression. Then we need to draw a line in the sand and take a stand against the Evil One. After all, he is just a big bully like Goliath the Philistine. We can take him down by using the sword of God's Word.

> *Be self-controlled and alert. Your enemy the devil prowls around like a roaring lion looking for someone to devour. Resist him, standing firm in the faith, because you know that your brothers throughout the world are undergoing the same kind of sufferings.* —1 Peter 5:8-9

Shrugging off the Stigma

Unfortunately, there is often a huge stigma attached to mental illness. In the beginning I found it a bit of a challenge to tell others that I had been booked into a psychiatric hospital. However, my experience at AKESO was a great eye-opener and radically changed my perceptions. It was not an institution for handling and treating those with serious mental disorders, but rather a safe place where those, mentally mauled by the hardships of this world, could recuperate.

I met all sorts of people at AKESO, normal people from all walks of life, but people struggling with problems that had become too much for them to handle alone. Some suffered depression and had even attempted suicide, whilst others had to work through the terrible heartache of divorce. There were those who had suffered both physical and mental abuse at the hands of family members, whilst others had gone through rehab recently to overcome substance abuse.

I was happy to be simply one of the crowd and to listen to people's stories, but I soon found that I was offering comfort and counsel to a number of people. I was aware that God was using me as a kind of "broken healer". Somehow, other inmates found it easy to approach me as a pastor in a psychiatric hospital because I was "in the same boat" as they were. I found I was more compassionate and better able to identify with the problems; others were grappling with. I have fond memories of this time I spent as one of the mentally bruised and broken and believe that it was a necessary pit stop in my journey through life with Jesus.

Lessons Learnt

- Prayer should be exercised as a form of teamwork between the believer and the Holy Spirit.

- We should not be afraid of expressing emotions in prayer since Jesus did so during his earthly ministry.

- The major changes that cancer sometimes brings in our lives can evoke a spirit of mourning and lead to depression.

- Sometimes we first have to pass through a time of sorrow or weeping before we can enter into our future joy.

- We do not have to perform in order to earn or win God's love and acceptance. We simply need to receive His forgiveness and fatherly embrace and to revel in our identity as children of God.

- Depression can be a form of spiritual oppression which needs to be fought with spiritual weapons. A believer has authority to break the bondage of depression in Jesus' name.

- We should not put up with mental confusion but claim the fact that God has given us a sound mind.

Key Facts

- Cancer patients sometimes have to fight infections which may result in high fevers. High fevers and insomnia in turn may result in delirium.

- Sometimes the cause of depression is a physical condition like biochemical or hormonal imbalances in the body. Hypothyroidism is one such condition.

Notes

1. Drugs.com 2020. Carfilzomib. Online article at URL:https://www.drugs.com/cdi/carfilzomib.html Accessed 2020-08-14

Chapter 14

Five Stones for the Fight

In the historical record of David taking on the giant Goliath we read the following:

Then he [David] took his staff in his hand, chose five smooth stones from the stream, put them in the pouch of his shepherd's bag and, with his sling in his hand, approached the Philistine. —1 Samuel 17:40

Reaching into his bag and taking out a stone, he slung it and struck the Philistine on the forehead. The stone sank into his forehead, and he fell face down on the ground. —1 Samuel 17:49

It's remarkable that with a single stone from his sling, David was able to fell the giant. Of course, it was not so much the stone which gave him the victory but his implicit trust in the God of Israel and his courageous faith which galvanised him into action.

As you face your giant called Cancer, there are five "stones" I'd like to recommend you put in your pouch and include in your armoury. All five are important and will ensure you employ a holistic, multi-pronged approach to defeating this disease. Each of the five will be rendered more effective should you have an underlying trust in God as your ultimate physician.

We must pursue wholeness and health holistically, understanding that we are tripartite beings made up of spirit, soul and body and that the different dimensions of our being are interdependent. The apostle John began one of his letters with a prayer for his friend Gaius which is insightful: *Dear friend, I pray that you may enjoy good health and that all may go well with you, even as your soul is getting along well.* **(3 John 1:2)** He implies that good health and the wellbeing of the soul are co-dependent.

The Stone of Faith

There are many who take the view that having a "positive attitude" will help you in your fight against cancer, but there are also detractors who disagree. Cancer patients sometimes complain of well-meaning family and friends who encourage them to think positively and keep their chins up when they have neither the mental nor the emotional capacity for this. This can add to their emotional stress and they can begin to feel that nobody really understands what they are going through leading to a sense of isolation. Faith is more than pasting on a happy face and pretending you are okay when inside you are falling apart.

As I said earlier in my chapter on the fight of faith, there is a huge difference between merely thinking positively and believing in God. Trying to cultivate a positive mind-set in the face of discouraging facts can end up being a fruitless and frivolous mental exercise. No! Faith needs a focus! We need to deposit our trust in something solid; our faith needs a firm foundation in something, someone outside ourselves. Someone bigger and more powerful than us, someone wiser than we are, someone willing to help. What better foundation than to believe in the goodness, the compassion, the love and the mercy of a God who wants us to call him Father. There are certain things we need to believe about God in order to have a sure faith. I'd like to mention a few since our faith needs to have content in order for it to be well-rounded and well-founded.

Firstly, since we are fighting a giant of a disease called Cancer, we need to be convinced that it is God's will to heal. Our Father has revealed His will in His Word. Not only did He introduce himself to us as Jehovah Rophe – the God who heals and give us many promises of healing, but He also sent his Son Jesus to be the Living Word, a full and complete revelation of who He is and what He stands for. If we follow the public ministry of Jesus as recorded in the Gospels, we are confronted with healing after healing, miracle after miracle, page after page. Although Jesus is now at the right hand of the Father in heaven, He has not changed. *Jesus Christ is the same yesterday and today and forever.* **(Hebrews 13:8)** I believe it is still His will to heal the sick.

Perhaps you believe that God Almighty has the power to heal but you are not yet convinced if He is indeed willing to heal you. This incident in the ministry of Jesus will hopefully convince you that God is both willing and able to heal you: *A man with leprosy came to him and begged him on his knees, "If you are willing, you can make me clean." Filled with compassion, Jesus reached out his hand and touched the man. "I am willing," he said. "Be clean!" Immediately the leprosy left him and he was cured.* **(Mark 1:40-42)**

Notice that the man believed that Jesus could heal him but was not sure if He were willing to, hence the pleading. Jesus was visibly moved with compassion and demonstrated His love by touching the untouchable leper and then pronounced, *"I am willing, be clean!"* I'm convinced God is willing and loves to heal the sick. Sometimes He does so immediately; other times healing is a process, but He's still in the healing business.

Another thing we need to be convinced of is the unfailing love of God. Love is a central attribute of God; God is love. We need to have faith in God's everlasting love. *...we know and rely on the love God has for us. God is love. Whoever lives in love lives in God, and God in him.* **(1 John 4:16).** People who are sure of God's love are not tossed about by circumstances, but can ride the storms of life. Although the Apostle Paul went through many trials and tribulations and faced much persecution, he did not doubt the love of God and was able to state the following with conviction:

No, in all these things we are more than conquerors through him who loved us. For I am convinced that neither death nor life, neither angels nor demons, neither the present nor the future, nor any powers, neither height nor depth, nor anything else in all creation, will be able to separate us from the love of God that is in Christ Jesus our Lord. **(Romans 8:37-39).** What about you? Are you convinced of the love of God?

Another important component of a sure faith is to believe in the Word of God and the promises of God. God watches over His Word to perform it. **(Jeremiah 1:12)**. God's Word will not return to Him empty, but will accomplish the purpose for which He sent it. **(Isaiah 55:11).** God keeps His covenant of love and does not fail to deliver on His promises. The prophet Balaam made this statement and asked this question: *God is not a man, that he should lie, nor a son of man, that he should change his mind. Does he speak and then not act? Does he promise and not fulfil?* **(Numbers 23:19)**

In this age of fear and uncertainty as we live on a polluted planet in the grip of global warming and in the claws of a Corona virus pandemic, it's good to know that God's Word will outlive even the created order. Jesus affirmed this, saying *Heaven and earth will pass away, but my words will never pass away.* **(Mark 13:31)**

So why don't you pick up this stone of faith? It will help you to fight off doubt and fear and to appropriate healing in spite of what the medical reports may say. God is not confined to or regulated by the opinions of man. He is ...*the God who gives life to the dead and calls things that are not as though they were.* **(Romans 4:17)** He can call us healed when we have been pronounced sick. *We accept man's testimony, but*

God's testimony is greater because it is the testimony of God... **(1 John 5:9)**

Faith throws open the door to incredible opportunity. In fact, Jesus said. *"Everything is possible for him who believes."* *(Mark 9:23) Do you* want to be victorious as you go against Goliath? Do you want to be a world overcomer? *Everyone born of God overcomes the world. This is the victory that has overcome the world, even our faith.* **(1 John 5:4)**

The Stone of Prayer

One of the ways of putting faith into action is through prayer. Prayer brings God onto the scene and when God pitches up things happen. Andrew Murray apparently said, *"When man works – he works! When man prays – God works".* Do you want to get God working on your behalf? Well, you know what to do!

The Scriptures are laced with many invitations for us to pray. In His Sermon on the Mount Jesus urged the eager crowd to pray saying, *"Ask and it will be given to you; seek and you will find; knock and the door will be opened to you. For everyone who asks receives; he who seeks finds; and to him who knocks, the door will be opened.* **(Matthew 7:7-8)** He issued another personal invitation to His disciples shortly before going to the cross saying, *"...I tell you the truth, my Father will give you whatever you ask in my name. Until now you have not asked for anything in my name. Ask and you will receive, and your joy will be complete.* **(John 16:23-24)** How scandalous it would be to ignore such open invitations and to stumble through life's problems and hurdles unaided! How scathing to hear these words of accusation, *"...You do not have, because you do not ask God."* **(James 4:2)**

Prayer is a wonderful privilege believers have. How awesome it is to have an audience with Almighty God, to be able to enter the courts of heaven in prayer and come before His throne with our requests, prayers and supplication. Since Jesus our high priest has gone before us, *"Let us then approach the throne of grace with confidence, so that we may receive mercy and find grace to help us in our time of need."* **(Hebrews 4:16)**. To help you along I have included some example prayers in previous chapters. I would urge you to use them merely as a guideline and to personalise them if possible.

I also mentioned that I had elicited the prayers of others as well and would encourage you to do the same. There were times in my battles with cancer that I did not have the capacity for prayer other than to whisper the words: "Help me Jesus!" At such times I believe that I was literally carried along by the prayers of others. In order to keep these "prayer warriors" informed I created a WhatsApp broadcast group and from time to time would give some feedback on my progress or ask for specific prayers when facing a challenge. Together we knocked on the doors of heaven and were answered by a living, loving God.

Why don't you try asking, seeking and knocking through prayer? Don't fail to add this stone to your pouch.

The Stone of Eating Right

To eat or not to eat – that is the question!

When people are aware that you are fighting cancer, they tend to bombard you with all sorts of good advice on what you should or shouldn't be eating. There are also the miracle ingredients or herbal cures which they insist, if people would only take, would reduce the prevalence of cancer in a jiffy. All this can be both confusing and a bit tiresome. Heck, if I'd taken all this seriously, I would have been eating grated lemon peels, munching grape seeds, drinking epsom salts, lacing my food with cayenne pepper and avoiding all sugar etc. One has to take it all with a pinch of salt and just smile and say, "Thanks for the advice." Or "I'll read the article." Or "I'll watch the video".

Be discerning about this kind of information. Most of these remedies are only supported by anecdotal claims and have not been scientifically tested. Unfortunately, the internet is a fertile breeding ground for enthusiastically communicated, unproven theories.

That said, I must point out that I have been taking a daily shot of turmeric, black pepper, cinnamon, lemon juice and honey almost continuously for the past three years (Recipe in Appendix 2). I was careful to inform my physicians of this and was advised not to take it during my stem-cell transplant. (This was simply to avoid the complication of any unknown interactions between the herbal remedy and the chemotherapy drugs). I consider turmeric to be the most important ingredient in the mix. For centuries it has been considered by Asian nations to have medicinal properties. It is a potent natural anti-inflammatory. It also has anti-bacterial properties and promotes intestinal health. I believe it helps prevent mucositis (inflammation in the mouth, throat and intestines); something which is common for cancer patients on chemotherapy. I have never suffered from these side-effects. There is also anecdotal evidence that turmeric can play a positive role in the treatment of certain cancers including multiple myeloma.

I believe that diet plays a supportive role in helping us fight cancer, rather than being the cure. It is unlikely that components of our diet can reverse genetic mutations in cancer cells. They can, however, help boost our immune response and supply vital ingredients for the production of the various categories of blood cells by our bone marrow. This is especially important for cancer patients on chemotherapy as cell multiplication in their bone marrow is invariably retarded. This being the case, I would advise eating an iron rich diet. Iron is an essential component of haemoglobin, the oxygen carrying molecule prevalent in our red blood cells. Dark green vegetables like spinach, broccoli and kale are rich in iron as are liver, red meat and sar-

141

dines. Vitamin B9 (folic acid) also aids the uptake of iron by our digestive system. If you are taking an iron tablet/capsule, try to ensure that it has iron in the form of a chelate and that it also includes folic acid. Vitamin C boosts our immune system and aids the production of white blood cells which are essential in our immune response. I would advise eating vitamin C rich fruits like oranges, grapefruit, guavas and naartjies and perhaps boosting your vitamin C with a daily effervescent supplement.

Cancer cells multiply rapidly and have a high metabolic rate. As a result, they consume more energy than healthy cells and catabolise carbohydrates speedily. High levels of carbohydrates in the diet result in elevated blood sugar levels which could favour the growth of cancer cells. Bear in mind though, that healthy cells also need to catabolise sugar for energy. If one does not suffer from diabetes and exercises regularly, then a certain amount of sugar in the diet is essential otherwise one will end up being lethargic because of low blood sugar levels.

Although I have not totally eliminated my sugar intake, I have reduced it substantially. I still drink an energy rich sports hydration drink containing phosphates and electrolytes when I exercise. The exercise itself burns off the carbohydrate and free sugar in the mix. I have also reduced my caffeine intake substantially and often drink rooibos tea (redbush tea) instead of Ceylon tea or coffee. I add some ginger and sweeten it a bit with raw honey (See Appendix 3). Both the rooibos infusion and ginger have known healing properties. Of course, heavy drinking of alcohol and smoking is an anathema for cancer sufferers. Fortunately, I have never smoked cigarettes or consumed alcohol, so I have not had to discipline myself to curtail these habits. May God give you strength should you need to reduce your alcohol consumption or quit smoking!

But enough said, the various cancer websites have much good advice on diet should you require further information. (See appendix)

I hope I've convinced you about the importance of eating a healthy diet if you are fighting cancer and that you are ready to add this stone to your armoury.

The Stone of Regular Exercise

To sweat or not to sweat – that is also a question!

I have made a case for the benefit of exercise throughout the preceding chapters, so I will not belabour the point much here.

In summary, exercise stimulates our circulation and metabolism, helps eliminate toxins from the body, can accelerate our recovery and increase our longevity. Aerobic and anaerobic exercises stimulate the production of haemoglobin and the manufacture of red blood cells and therefore can help prevent anaemia, a common problem with cancer patients. It's a known fact that many long-term cancer survivors exercise regularly and are therefore physically fit.

I try to exercise five times a week and vary my program between swimming (in the summer months), vigorous walking, cycling, jogging, and gym exercises. A good exercise session results in the release of "happy endorphins" and gives one a sense of well-being. It is a good antidote for depression which dogs many cancer sufferers. Sure, exercise requires some commitment and self-discipline, but as I've said before, "Cancer isn't for sissies!"

Some consider me a bit of a fitness fanatic, so don't mind me. You must find an exercise program that works for you. It is better to start small and build things up gradually than to be too ambitious when you start exercising. A small amount of exercise on a regular basis pays better dividends than over exerting yourself once a fortnight.

One of the best ways of keeping yourself going is to exercise with a friend or two. That way you can hold each other mutually accountable. You can also track your progress on a smartphone or sports watch and report your achievements on an app like Strava or Samsung health.

Are you ready to join me in the swimming pool? Why don't you dive in and add the stone of physical exercise to your arsenal?

The Stone of Self-Advocacy

Self-advocacy means taking charge of your care. It involves asking lots of questions, understanding the type of cancer you have and doing some reading and self-study so that you have a good grasp of the enemy you're fighting. I have heard patients say that they have absolute faith in their physician's judgment and that they don't even know what drugs are in their drips. Besides, they add, they really don't understand all the medical jargon anyway. They say that "ignorance is bliss", but I believe that people perish for a lack of knowledge. *(See Hosea 4:6)*. Fortunately, I have the advantage of a scientific background which helps me understand some of the jargon and with that I have an enquiring mind that just needs to know the detail of the how, the why and the wherefore. I have found that most doctors appreciate someone who respectfully asks questions, even the occasional dumb ones. I have found that being "in the know" has helped me have a sense of control even in difficult and uncertain times.

Although I consider faith in a healing God to be of primary importance, I also believe in tapping into the best treatment procedures that humankind has on offer. So, I'm all in for the best both heaven and earth can provide. Cancer research continues apace and as a result new and better treatment protocols are continually being developed and introduced. Unfortunately, some of the newest treatment options are also the most expensive, so financial considerations may influence the decisions as to which treatment route to follow.

Medical practitioners are fallible human beings and not all of them stay informed of the latest developments in oncology and therefore not all treatment centres are on a par. Before one commits to a certain physician or institution one will do well to ask some questions about what treatment option they would propose. Try to find out more about their success rate and also weigh up the pros and cons of the treatment on offer. Of course, it will be good to get one or two different opinions before you make a final decision if that is at all possible.

Self-advocacy doesn't end with the initial treatment choice but continues right through to the decisions around follow-up care after treatment. Although I've been in remission for some time I'm still informed and will be personally involved in the process of deciding what treatment to use should the need arise. I am still in touch with the latest research being done on treating MM and I keep my health team on their toes by asking difficult questions. What about you, have you done any reading and self-study about your particular disease? Could you tell me on what treatment you are and why? They say that knowledge is power and I believe that to be true. Why don't you begin to play an active role in your treatment? After all, it's your own body which is on the line! Why don't you select the stone of self-advocacy?

CHAPTER 15

A BALANCED BATTLE PLAN

One of the difficulties many Christian believers face is how to balance faith in God with some of the practical decisions and actions we have to take in life, especially when it comes to availing ourselves of medical help. In my pastoral ministry I have had to grapple with these "issues of faith" both personally as well as in trying to give wise, Biblical counsel to my church members. They were also brought into more sharp focus by my personal battles with cancer. These "issues of faith" are often behind some of the difficult questions believers ask.

In this chapter I'd like to address a few pertinent questions which may have arisen in your mind as you've engaged in the fight against cancer or as you've supported friends or family members in their battle against the disease. I believe we need to answer these questions if we are to come up with a balanced battle plan. What I say may challenge some of your personal or religious convictions, but I would urge you to hear me out before coming to a conclusion.

How Does One Balance the Natural and the Supernatural?

The Gospels are replete with accounts of the miracles, signs and wonders that attended Jesus' public ministry. Many of the miracles were instantaneous healings of various diseases. To me, to believe in Jesus is to believe in the supernatural power of God. The question which arises in my mind and the minds of many is this: "If I indeed believe in divine healing, then why would I need to seek out the help of human physicians?" I have already attempted to answer this question early on in this book (in Chapter 2) when I spoke about faith and the use of medicines, but since it is such an important question that begs an answer, I will try to answer it from a different perspective here.

Many reading this book probably come from a Western background as I do. We need to realise that our Western world view has been strongly influenced by Greek thought. Greek philosophers tended to bring a sharp divide between the material and the spiritual. Matter was regarded as evil whilst spirit was deemed good. As a result, the physical body was regarded as evil and was seen to be the prison of the soul. In Greek thought there was/is therefore a deep disconnect between the secular and the spiritual, the natural and the supernatural. (This is not the case in Hebrew, African and Eastern thought. In these different cultures everything is deemed to be deeply spiritual.)

If we are under the influence of Western thought, we tend to subconsciously compartmentalise our lives into the secular and the spiritual. For example, when we are praying, we believe we are doing something spiritual, whereas when we are eating, that's not spiritual at all. If we are in church, we see ourselves as being engaged in spiritual things, whilst when we are at work, we are busy with our secular jobs. We introduce an artificial separation, a false dichotomy between the secular and the spiritual. This is not supposed to be the case. From a Biblical perspective everything is deemed to be of spiritual significance:

And whatever you do, whether in word or deed, do it all in the name of the Lord Jesus, giving thanks to God the Father through him. —Colossians 3:17

A Balanced Battle Plan

***Whatever you do, work at it with all your heart, as
working for the Lord, not for men, since you know
that you will receive an inheritance from the Lord
as a reward. It is the Lord Christ you are serving.***
—Colossians 3:23-24

We tend to bring this idea into our approach towards
health and healing. To pray and ask God to heal us "supernaturally" is spiritual, whereas consulting a doctor is
very "unspiritual" – it is seen to be seeking worldly advice
and help. I must, however, ask the question, "Is it not possible that God may answer our prayer for healing by direct-
ing us to a physician whom He has gifted with a
knowledge and understanding of medicine?" If we are only
open to a so-called "supernatural healing," are we not dic-
tating to God the method we expect Him to use? Let us
not limit God to our human expectations!

I certainly believe that we should first go to God with
our need for healing since He is the ultimate healer. The
other day I read this interesting Scripture which underlines
this: *In the thirty-ninth year of his reign Asa was afflicted with a
disease in his feet. Though his disease was severe, even in his illness he
did not seek help from the LORD, but only from the physicians.* (**2
Chronicles 16:12**). The real problem was not that Asa
sought help from the physicians, but that he did so exclu-
sively without seeking help from the LORD Yahweh.

When we think of Jesus and the "supernatural", let us
consider a few things:

On one occasion Jesus surprised, even frightened his
disciples by walking on water. (***See John 6:19***). However,
he normally crossed the Sea of Galilee by sailing in a fish-
ing boat. In fact, on one occasion he even borrowed
Simon and Andrew's boat as a preaching platform. (***See
Luke 5:3***). Why didn't He simply stand on the water?
Surely that would have impressed the crowd?! On two
occasions Jesus miraculously multiplied bread and fish to

feed the five thousand (*See Matthew 14:15-21*) and the four thousand. (*Matthew 15:38*). However, his disciples normally obtained food by purchasing it from the nearest town. (*John 4:8*). My point is that Jesus usually followed the normal, expected order of things. However, on occasion he displayed his divine power by overriding the natural order and doing something we label "supernatural". I don't want to make a rule of this, but Jesus seemed to do this when there was no "natural" way to solve the problem. He was alone praying on a mountain and there was no boat to ferry him to his disciples so he walked on the water. In both instances of supernatural provision of food, the crowds had followed him to remote places where no food was available so Jesus provided food miraculously.

I was greatly helped when, as a young Christian, I heard a medical Doctor, who believed in divine healing, share the following insights:

When Jesus went to the tomb of Lazarus, He didn't wave his arms to remove the stone miraculously. Human help was available so he asked some men to remove the stone. Then, he did what was humanly impossible; he cried out, "Lazarus, come forth!" and Lazarus arose miraculously from the tomb. Following that, he instructed some standers-by to unbind Lazarus' grave clothes. Again, human help was available so Jesus did not unbind Lazarus miraculously, but followed a natural approach. (*See John 11:38-45*). In this way the natural and the supernatural interacted in the raising of Lazarus.

In the same way God can employ natural human means and combine them with his divine intervention to do something we would label miraculous or supernatural. He can use your physician and the medicine prescribed, but then add his "super" to the "natural" help they provide to do something "supernatural." Therefore, I would advocate a balanced approach to healing and health. I would seek the best help that modern medicine can provide, but at the same time anticipate that the immortal God can break into the realm of our mortality in response to our faith and in answer to our prayers. Let us have faith in a merciful, healing God as we employ even natural means to obtain healing and health.

If I Trust in God for My Health, Why Would I Need Medical Insurance?

There are many wonderful promises of both provision and protection in the Word of God. For instance, Jesus encouraged his followers not to worry about what they would eat or drink or about what they would wear, but to consider the lilies of the field and the birds of the air and how God clothed them and fed them. **(*See Matthew 6:25-33*)**. One of my favourite Scriptures which promises provision reads: *And God is able to make all grace abound to you, so that in all things at all times, having all that you need, you will abound in every good work.* **(2 Corinthians 9:8)**. (Note the repetition of the words *abound* and *all*. I have memorised this Scripture and declare it over my life frequently).

When it comes to protection against danger and disease, perhaps some of the clearest promises are found in Psalm 91. Some even call it "the protection Psalm". Here are the first few verses:

> *He who dwells in the shelter of the Most High will rest in the shadow of the Almighty. I will say of the LORD, "He is my refuge and my fortress, my God, in whom I trust." Surely he will save you from the fowler's snare and from the deadly pestilence. He will cover you with his feathers, and under his wings you will find refuge; his faithfulness will be your shield and rampart. You will not fear the terror of night, nor the arrow that flies by day, nor the pestilence that stalks in the darkness, nor the plague that destroys at midday. A thousand*

may fall at your side, ten thousand at your right hand, but it will not come near you. —Psalm 91:1-7

This Psalm has been a wonderful source of reassurance to me and to many even as I write during the Covid-19 pandemic of 2020.

With the above in mind, many consider it to be an expression of a lack of trust and a waste of money if one takes out medical insurance. Shouldn't we simply just trust God for our health and our protection? In attempting to answer this conundrum, I'd like to refer you to two interesting and somewhat conflicting instructions that Jesus gave his disciples as he commissioned them for action. The first instruction was given when Jesus commissioned 72 of his followers to go ahead of him into the towns and villages he was later to visit: *Go! I am sending you out like lambs among wolves. Do not take a purse or bag or sandals; and do not greet anyone on the road...* **(Luke 10:3-4)**

Sometime later, just before Jesus was about to die on the Cross, he first asked his disciples a question and then changed his instructions radically: *Then Jesus asked them, "When I sent you without purse, bag or sandals, did you lack anything?" "Nothing," they answered. He said to them, "But now if you have a purse, take it, and also a bag; and if you don't have a sword, sell your cloak and buy one. It is written: 'And he was numbered with the transgressors'; and I tell you that this must be fulfilled in me. Yes, what is written about me is reaching its fulfilment." The disciples said, "See, Lord, here are two swords." "That is enough," he replied.* **(Luke 22:35-38)**

To me the purse and the sword speak of provision and protection. The disciples had lacked neither as they had gone out on previous missions. Now, however, the times were changing and persecution and danger were to be expected, hence Jesus' instruction to take both a purse and a sword or two along with them to ensure both provision and protection. I have gone through a similar experience in my own walk with the Lord…

As a young pastor working to grow and establish our church I had to "walk by faith" and trust God to provide for my family. We never lacked for anything, but at times things were tough and we had to work very carefully with our finances. The package which the church leadership offered me included medical insurance for me and my family. However, for a time during the building of the first phase of our church facilities, the church was somewhat cash-strapped. As I prayed about this I sensed the Holy Spirit leading me to forego the protection and provision that the medical aid portfolio offered and to trust God for the health of my family.

I discussed this with my church leadership group and although they were a bit reticent to do so, I asked them to cancel our medical insurance until further notice. This would free more funds to be used for our building project. Thankfully there were enough finances to complete the building project. In spite of the project's completion, I continued for several years afterwards without the need for medical insurance by simply trusting in God for health and healing for my family. However, there came a time when I began to get an urgency in my spirit to re-instate a medical insurance policy which we then did.

I am so grateful that I was obedient to the Holy Spirit's promptings because the operations and treatments for my various cancer challenges would have ruined us financially had we not acquired medical insurance. I'm also quite sure we would have had to rule out some of the best treatment options because of financial constraints.

Cancer doesn't just impact one individual, but can impact on the whole family. I have a young man in our church whose sister contracted brain cancer when they were both still children. Their father was self-employed and ran a successful business. However, he had no medical insurance in place. Being a loving father, he spared no expense to get treatment for his ailing daughter. Because he was so preoccupied with getting help for his daughter, he ended up losing his business as well. Sadly, the young girl eventually died and the surviving family was left financially destitute and ended up living in a caravan. As a young boy, the son was placed in a boarding school hostel. He vividly recalls some of the hardships that he and his family went through as a result of his sister's illness. We need to be wise stewards of the finances which the Lord entrusts into our hands and protect ourselves against the thief who comes to rob, kill and destroy. *(See John 10:10).* We need to do what is humanly possible to guard ourselves against life's sometimes harsh eventualities whilst at the same time trusting in God for our provision and protection.

Isn't Treatment with Chemotherapy or Radiation Worse than the Disease Itself?

I've heard this question asked on a number of occasions. There is the perception that cancer treatment is horrible and unbearable. As a result, many refuse any treatment at all and choose to simply "trust God." Although this approach seems commendable it is sometimes motivated more by fear and ignorance than true faith. Others, often influenced by unverified information posted on the internet, choose to go the "natural route" and focus on diet and natural remedies instead. Unfortunately, the track records of both approaches are not that encouraging.

This example illustrates what I'm saying:

One day in the "chemo room" whilst I was on a drip, I struck up a conversation with a woman who had recently been diagnosed with breast cancer. She mentioned that she had five different friends or acquaintances who over time had all been diagnosed with breast cancer. Four had refused treatment and had chosen the "natural route", whilst one had undergone chemotherapy. Of the five, the woman who received treatment was the only one still alive. My newfound friend had a young family and for their sakes and on the grounds of what she had seen through the example of her friends, had wisely decided to submit to treatment. Like many other cancers, breast cancer is very treatable, especially if caught early, and many have lived to tell the tale.

In days gone by some cancer treatments were indeed pretty horrific. This is what gave rise to the perception we are confronting. However, ongoing cancer research is resulting in better and better drugs and treatment protocols. The drugs being used nowadays often have fewer side-effects than those of yesteryear, so to simply assume that the treatment is going to be worse than the disease itself is often to act in ignorance. I experienced very few side-effects during most of my treatment. Sure, there were times when things got tough, especially during my stem cell transplant when I was subjected to high dose chemotherapy, but on the whole I was able to enjoy good quality of life in the two and a half years I was receiving chemo. Heaven knows if I would still be alive or what suffering I would have had to endure if the disease were allowed to take its course.

It's a Question of Balance

The book of Proverbs, which is full of wise sayings, often exalts a prudent and sensible approach to life. If we are to triumph in this battle against this giant called cancer, I believe it would be prudent for us to have a balanced battle plan. Let us see no artificial divide between the natural and the spiritual. Let us be wise and insure ourselves against the sometimes-harsh realities we must face in life, realising that medical treatment can be very expensive. Finally, if we have the possibility and the privilege of receiving medical treatment, let us embrace the best that medical science can offer and combine it with the healing mercy that flows from the very heart of God.

CHAPTER 16

A SEASON OF PEACE

Fortunately, in this long war of attrition against cancer, the battle waxes and wanes. There are seasons of intense warfare, but there are thankfully also seasons of peace. In the oncology department of the hospital or in the chemo room, one encounters people in different phases of their individual battles against the enemy. Some appear a bit haggard and war-weary, whilst others in remission are full of the joys of spring. As I write I am fortunate to find myself in a season of peace.

Battling Back to Zero

During my season in AKESO, my psychiatrist was able to rule out the possibility of my mental state being the result of my treatment with Kyprolis. Both the MRI of my brain and the EEG ruled out the possibility that I was suffering from PRES which, as I've said, is a very rare but dangerous side-effect of the drug. With this valuable information in hand, my oncologist was able to continue my treatment using a combination of Kyprolis and Dexamethazone, abbreviated Kd.

I had imported enough Kyprolis for three cycles of treatment. Each cycle involved three weekly infusions of Kyprolis and Dexamethazone at the chemo room in Nelspruit. I would then have a week's respite from all drugs before beginning the next 21-day cycle. Before each cycle I would have full blood tests including serum electrophoresis to determine my M-protein score.

Going Against Goliath

We made steady progress in the battle back to zero and progressed from an M score of two down to zero over the next three months. Whether it was the Kyprolis or the combination of the drug with dexamethasone that brought down my count, no-one will really know. I believe that much of the progress was the product of faith-energised prayer. I experienced minimal side-effects during this time except that I was rather hyped up by the weekly dose of steroids which required me to take a sleeping tablet for two nights of the week.

One interesting side-effect of the steroid was that it promoted hair growth, so it wasn't long before my bald head was transformed into a mop of dark wavy hair. A few people commented that I looked younger than I had before when my hair had been a steely grey in colour. I also took the opportunity of sporting a beard, something I'd never done before in my life. This sure got the tongues of the ladies in our congregation wagging and particularly impressed some of the younger folk. What one has to do to keep people interested in your sermons!

I had a trivalent flu vaccine before winter and I am taking careful precautions against infection during the current Covid-19 pandemic. I rejoice that as I write I have been in full remission for the past nine months but realise that I may still have to fight further battles. There are many MM veterans who are a lot further down the road than I am. The overall 5-year survival rate for people with multiple myeloma is currently 54% (Cancer.net 2020). My first diagnosis was only three years ago so it is still early days for me; I have not even reached the 5-year landmark yet. I hesitate to claim that I am healed. I did so for the eleven months after my stem cell transplant only to be humbled and disappointed by a spectacular relapse. Rather than being presumptuous I continue in faith believing that time will validate my healing.

I Preach for a Final Quarter

My relapse, hospitalisations, infection and subsequent mental battles meant that I was unable to preach for a period of about three months. I then had the privilege of returning to the pulpit for the last quarter of 2019 to preach a final series of messages before my retirement on 31 December 2019. During this last quarter we held a special farewell service where I symbolically passed the baton to my young associate pastor, Hein Vermaak, who has now succeeded me as senior pastor. It was a great occasion and the church was packed with people. I naturally experienced mixed emotions. There was a sense of fulfilment and accomplishment at having led and built up the church over 34 years; kind of like a mountain top experience. But, at the same time there was sadness at having to say goodbye to our precious church family and leave our amazing church facilities to others to steward. It is not easy to let go of your life's work without a sense of loss. The occasion ended with refreshments, eats and fellowship in true Living Waters style.

There were also other handovers and farewells. I had been the provincial leader of our church network TCN for several years and in that capacity had been overseeing some 30 churches in the province of Mpumalanga. It was also time for me to leave this work to a successor. The choice of the right candidate was easy and I was able to give over the reins to a great man of God, Pastor RD Kgatle, who has the DNA of TCN and a proven track record. Desi and I met with RD and his wife Anna and our other Regional Leaders for a farewell luncheon where they expressed their appreciation for the work we had done and where we were able to encourage them to continue building God's kingdom in our province and our land.

Where to from Here?

I have been retired now for nearly 10 months. My retirement has spelled the end of my regular pastoral and preaching responsibilities and has been accompanied by a sense of relief. Desi and I never realised what a weight of responsibility leading a church entailed until we were released from it. It's great for us to wake in the morning and to be able to pursue some of our own dreams. One of my goals has always been to start writing books and this is my first project; I hope you have enjoyed reading it. I trust there will be many more to follow. I also sense God calling me into an apostolic ministry of encouraging and empowering pastors of grassroots, rural churches.

Because of the Covid-19 pandemic there has been little movement in the property market and our plans to relocate to Pretoria have been put on hold. We are content to wait on the timing of God and in the interim we are still in Sabie playing an active role in our church as it navigates the Covid-19 lockdown. I still preach from time to time and lead worship every third week, but it is before video cameras rather than a live audience; a totally new experience! Who knows, perhaps I will exercise some of my apostolic calling through the medium of videos?

New Mercies for Each New Morning

Wherever you find yourself in your battle with cancer, whether it's in a time of intense warfare or in a season of peace, I want to encourage you never to give up hope and to keep fighting the good fight of the faith. It is not merely a physical battle you are fighting, but one which has mental, emotional and spiritual dimensions to it as well. There will be mountain top experiences and there will also be valleys, but God will be with you no matter what. This disease may even change the direction of our lives but we must not let it rob us of our sense of destiny.

A portion of Scripture which has been with me for years and has often encouraged me is found in Lamentations 3:21-23 and reads: *...this I call to mind and therefore I have hope: Because of the LORD's great love we are not consumed, for his compassions never fail. They are new every morning; great is your faithfulness.*

Because of the Lord's great love, you will not be consumed. It is my prayer that you will experience His steadfast love, His great faithfulness and new mercies for each new morning you awake to continue the fight.

Notes

1. Cancer.net 2020. Multiple Myeloma: Statistics. Online article at URL: https://www.cancer.net/cancer-types/multiple-myeloma/statistics Accessed 2020-08-26

EPILOGUE

The other day a friend who is also fighting MM contacted me. His treatment has been far more gruelling than mine since he has kidney failure and has to face hours on a dialysis machine every second day. He had a successful stem cell transplant about two years ago and was about to go in for a much-needed kidney transplant when his myeloma suddenly relapsed. This spelt the end of any prospects of a kidney transplant for at least the next two years and he is again on a rigorous chemotherapy regimen to bring the relapse under control.

My friend was absolutely devastated and was facing a crisis of faith. He was asking the question, "Where is God in all of this?" and made the comment, "I've trusted Him all along only to have my hopes dashed to the ground." Perhaps you too are asking the same kind of questions and going through the same emotions as you try to gather yourself following some or other setback in your treatment? How can I comfort and console you? How can I fan your flickering faith into flame once more?

He's Been There

In my darkest hours I have found great comfort in knowing that my Saviour Jesus Christ has already experienced all the hardships, the disappointments and the pain that this world can throw at us. As a result, He can identify with us fully in our own weakness, suffering and human frailty. *For we do not have a high priest who is unable to sympathize with our weaknesses, but we have one who has been tempted in every way, just as we are—yet was without sin.* **(Hebrews 4:15)**. Because he

163

himself suffered when he was tempted, he is able to help those who are being tempted. **(Hebrews 2:18)**

Jesus fought a lonely battle of the soul as He agonised in prayer in Gethsemane before he drank the cup of suffering on the Cross. Whilst his three closest disciples slept he battled on alone. Three times he fell with his face to the ground and prayed, *"My Father, if it is possible, may this cup be taken from me. Yet not as I will, but as you will."* **(Matthew 26:39).** However, it was indeed the Father's will that he should suffer as a guilt offering for our sins. *Yet it was the LORD's will to crush him and cause him to suffer…* **(Isaiah 53:10)** So, in obedience Jesus faced the sham of a trial, the lashing of the whip, the mockery of the soldiers and the jeers of the fickle crowd as he stumbled and dragged his cross to the hill called Calvary where they crucified him.

Have you experienced agonising pain as a nursing sister pierced you with a needle in search of a vein? Jesus knows your pain; after all, they nailed his hands and feet to the cross and then lifted it up. Have you felt dizzy and nauseous after receiving radiotherapy or chemotherapy? Jesus has been there; his lungs deprived of oxygen, he felt faint, dizzy and nauseous as he died a slow death of suffocation. Have you felt a sense of loneliness and isolation as you've fought your personal battle? Judas betrayed Jesus, his disciples abandoned him and fled, Peter denied even knowing him, whilst the fickle crowd rejected him in favour of Barabbas. On the Cross it seemed as if even the Father had forsaken him. *…Jesus cried out in a loud voice, "Eloi, Eloi, lama sabachthani?"—which means, "My God, my God, why have you forsaken me?"* **(Matthew 27:46)** You are not alone in your battle; Jesus knows your pain and sorrow and will neither leave you nor forsake you.

What fills me with hope and faith for my health is the fact that, through the cross, Jesus defeated sin, sickness, disease, death and the Devil himself. There is far more than forgiveness of sins in Christ's substitutionary death on the cross. Amongst his many benefits there is also healing for our bodies and our souls: *Surely, he took up our infirmities and carried our sorrows, yet we considered him stricken by God, smitten by him, and afflicted. But he was pierced for our transgressions, he was crushed for our iniquities; the punishment that brought us peace was upon him, and by his wounds we are healed.* **(Isaiah 53:4-5)**

One day as I reflected on Mark's account of the crucifixion and marvelled at the price Jesus was willing to pay, I was inspired to write this poem:

We Will Never Cease to Praise You

Blessed Saviour, crowned with thorns

Object of the soldiers' scorn

Clothed in raiment fit for kings

Cruelly beaten for us all

We will never cease to praise You

It was for us, you did it all

Righteous blood for our redemption

To the cursed earth did fall

Stumbling t'ward a hill called Calv'ry

Bleeding for a world forlorn

Gentle hands that healed the leper

By cruel nails, crushed and torn

Going Against Goliath

We will never cease to praise You
'Twas for us You died alone
With Your lifeblood, paid our ransom
Slaves set free, returning home

Holy Lamb of God, our Saviour
With the lawless ones did die
Draws all mankind to His glory
Now that He is lifted high

I will never cease to praise You
'Twas for me you took the pain
Hanging bare 'twixt earth and heaven
Covered all my sin and shame

In borrowed tomb they laid your body
But it was for a short while
Sown in weakness, raised in glory
You reign supreme from throne on high

Jesus in Your Cross I glory
Boasting not in my own pride
Your trail of blood, this humbled sinner
To God's heart, doth surely guide

Epilogue

The Ball is in Your Court

Throughout this book I have referred to my personal faith in the God of the Bible and have quoted numerous scriptures from His Word. If you are already a believer in Christ His Son, I trust that these verses have strengthened your faith and that my testimony has encouraged you to "keep fighting the good fight of the faith" as you battle cancer. However, if you have not yet "sealed the deal" and invited Christ into your life to be your Lord and Saviour, I don't want you to finish reading and to close this book without seriously considering making this life-changing decision which will also determine your eternal destiny.

None of us knows how much longer we have to live, not even the healthiest individual, let alone we who are fighting cancer. God forbid, but I could walk out into the street tomorrow and be run over by a truck. This life is a mere breath in the face of eternity. Whether we live for seventeen or for seventy years is of little consequence when compared to the extent of our potential existence for all eternity. For instance, if I were to lay down matchsticks end to end across the continent of Africa from Cape Town to Cairo, my temporal life on this earth would be no more in length than one matchstick in comparison with the length of the millions and millions of matchsticks crossing the continent which represent eternity.

We can potentially spend all of eternity in the glorious presence of God. Or we can reject God's offer of salvation in Christ and end up separated from Him for all eternity. The choice is ours. We read this description of the quality of life in heaven: *And I heard a loud voice from the throne saying, "Now the dwelling of God is with men, and he will live with them. They will be his people, and God himself will be with them and be their God. He will wipe every tear from their eyes. There will be no more death or mourning or crying or pain, for the old order of things has passed away." (Revelation 21:3-4).* I am looking forward to dwelling with God where there is no more death or mourning or crying or pain and no more cancer! How about you?

So, what steps should one take to be born into the family of God and to seal one's eternal destiny? Four verses in John's gospel put it very simply and clearly for us...

Born into God's Family

He was in the world, and though the world was made through him, the world did not recognize him. He came to that which was his own, but his own did not receive him. Yet to all who received him, to those who believed in his name, he gave the right to become children of God—children born not of natural descent, nor of human decision or a husband's will, but born of God. —John 1:10-13

But to all who believed Him and accepted Him, He gave the right to become children of God. They are reborn—not with a physical birth resulting from human passion or plan, but a birth that comes from God. —John 1:12-13 NLT

In this passage we see three key words which show us three ways we need to respond if we want to become children of God:

Firstly, I Need to Recognize Who Jesus Is

(10) He was in the world, and though the world was made through him, the world did not recognize him.

There was this problem that many failed to recognise who Jesus really was. Many still fail to recognise who Jesus was and is. They think he was just a prophet or a good man who lived long ago; that he was just one amongst many holy men who can lead us to God. Others think he deceived the people or he's a fairy tale or even a swear word. But, Jesus was God in the flesh; he was both fully human and fully divine at the same time.

God had to become a man in order to get through to humankind. He was high and lofty and holy and many held Him in awe, yet did not know Him at all. So, God took on human flesh and went to great lengths to reveal Himself to man, but unfortunately, many stumbled over the humanity of Jesus thinking – "He's just a man!" For instance, when Jesus visited and taught in his own boyhood town of Nazareth this is how the people reacted: *Everyone spoke well of Him and was amazed by the gracious words that came from His lips. "How can this be?" they asked. "Isn't this Joseph's son?"* **(Luke 4:22 NLT)**

They expressed both amazement and rejection in the same breath. *Matthew 13:57* says, *And they took offense at him.* But others from other towns in Galilee continued to follow Jesus, gobsmacked by the miracles he was doing. Of course, the 12 disciples stuck closely to Him and there came a day when Jesus asked them the question: ...*"Who do people say the Son of Man is?" They replied, "Some say John the Baptist; others say Elijah; and still others, Jeremiah or one of the prophets." "But what about you?" he asked. "Who do you say I am?" Simon Peter answered, "You are the Christ, the Son of the living God." Jesus replied, "Blessed are you, Simon son of Jonah, for this was not revealed to you by man, but by my Father in heaven.* **(Matthew 16:13-17)**

In that moment there was true recognition from Peter of who Jesus was and is. He recognised that Jesus was the Messiah sent from God; the Saviour that they had been waiting for. Jesus was elated and said, *flesh and blood did not reveal it to you, but my Father in heaven.*

However, another form of recognition also has to take place. Not only do I need to recognize that Jesus is the Saviour; I need to recognize that I have need of a Saviour. All of us need a Saviour whether we realise it or not: ... *for all have sinned and fall short of the glory of God.* **(Romans 3:23)** We need to come to the place of brokenness and humility where we cry out "Lord save me." If we do, we will be rescued. The Bible says that *"Everyone who calls on the name of the Lord will be saved."* **(Romans 10:13)**

So, in order to be saved, we must first recognize that Jesus is the Saviour and that we need saving.

Secondly, To Be Born into God's Family I Need to Believe in Jesus

(12) NLT But to all who believed Him and accepted Him, He gave the right to become children of God.

Many accept or "believe" that a famous man called Jesus lived some two thousand years ago. They nod their heads and say, "I know of this man called Jesus." You could call that mental assent; they acknowledge Jesus. However, this kind of head knowledge about Christ is not enough to save you. Even the devil and his demon cohorts know about Jesus, but this does them no good. *You believe that there is one God. Good! Even the demons believe that—and shudder.* **(James 2:19)**

For us to be rescued or redeemed a more profound kind of believing is needed. I want to call this "saving faith". *(12) But to all who believed Him and accepted Him, He gave the right to become children of God.*

> **For it is by grace you have been saved, through faith...** —Ephesians 2:8

I must believe and trust in such a way that I am willing to let go of my life and put it into the hands of God. I must 'let go and let God'. Jesus said, *...whoever wants to save his life will lose it, but whoever loses his life for me will save it.* **(Luke 9:24).**

Epilogue

It is easy to say that I believe a parachute will save me, but the acid test of that belief will come the day I'm in an aircraft and the engine cuts out and I have to take the leap of faith. Saving faith requires that I trust Jesus enough to take that leap of faith and cast my life into his loving hands. I must believe that he is the Son of God; the Saviour sent from God and that he came to seek and to save me; that he died for my sins and rose again on the third day. I must believe in the person of Jesus and in the work of Jesus. It has nothing to do with any good works that I try to do, but has everything to do with my believing in the finished work of Christ on the Cross. As a great man of God, Angus Buchan often says: *"Good people don't go to heaven; believers go to heaven!"*

Rom 10:9 ...if you confess with your mouth, "Jesus is Lord," and believe in your heart that God raised him from the dead, you will be saved.

Thirdly, to be Born into God's Family I Must Receive Jesus

(12) Yet to all who received him, to those who believed in his name, he gave the right to become children of God

To receive salvation, I must receive the Saviour into my life. It's logical but I can miss it. I can go in and out of church without ever coming to the point of inviting Jesus into my heart to be my Lord and Saviour. I can pray up a storm because of my cancer condition, but still hold God at arm's length. Say I was given the gift of a large amount of money; someone wrote out a cheque for $100 000 with my name on it. What if I ran into the bank waving the cheque around, dancing for joy and shouting, "Look at what a great gift I've been given!" and then ran out again? Would the gift help me in any way? No! Why? Because no transaction would have taken place. I would need to go to the teller and deposit the cheque into my account. Only then could I draw money and start enjoying the gift.

You see, many people have been in and out of church nearly all their lives, they've prayed prayers and done all sorts of religious stuff, but no spiritual transaction has ever taken place. They've never come to the place of depositing their sins at the foot of the Cross, asking Jesus' forgiveness and then inviting Him into their lives to be their Lord and Saviour.

It's only when we do this that we are reborn and become children of God. *(12) Yet to all who received him, to those who believed in his name, he gave the right to become children of God.* It's only when we receive the Son that we receive eternal life. *...God has given us eternal life, and this life is in his Son. He who has the Son has life; he who does not have the Son of God does not have life.* **(1 John 5:11-12)**

How do you receive Jesus into your life? He is not physically present, but He's here spiritually. Jesus is saying, *Here I am! I stand at the door and knock. If anyone hears my voice and opens the door, I will come in and eat with him, and he with me.* **(Revelation 3:20)**

If you want a relationship with Jesus, you must open the door of your heart in prayer and invite Him in. He's a gentleman, He won't force his way in; he will patiently knock and wait for your response. Is Jesus knocking at the door of your heart today? What will your response be?

To Become a Child of God Here Is What You Must Do:

1. Recognize who Jesus is

2. Believe and entrust your life to Him

3. Receive Jesus into your heart and life

A Prayer for Salvation

Father God, I thank you for sending your Son Jesus to this earth to seek and to save the lost. Thank you, Jesus, that you searched for me and have found me.

I believe that you died for my sins and rose again on the third day; that You have paid the price for my healing and for my salvation.

Please forgive my sin and my rebellion and come into my life today to be my Lord and Saviour. I entrust my life into your hands.

Thank you, Jesus, for hearing my prayer. I rejoice that today I have become a child of God. Amen.

If you just prayed this prayer for the first time, then your identity has changed; you are now a child of God. How wonderful is that! Something else also changed; your eternal destiny. You now have a secure future since you have received the gift of eternal life. Jesus explained it this way: *I tell you the truth, those who listen to My message and believe in God who sent Me have eternal life. They will never be condemned for their sins, but they have already passed from death into life.* **(John 5:24 NLT)**

Did you get that? You have eternal life; you have already passed from death into life. If this is the case, then you need have no fear of death. Death has lost its sting. Death is merely a transition into a more glorious form of being. Death will usher you into the very presence of Almighty God.

Walking in a relationship with God has benefits for us in this earthly life and prepares us for the heavenly life to come. We have a new quality of life; Jesus described it as abundant life *(See John 10:10)*. We have a new quantity of life; a life that goes on forever; eternal life. *(See John 3:16)*

I am convinced that I am not alone as I face the various challenges that come my way in this life and as I battle cancer; I know that God is with me and so I am at peace. When my journey in this world is done, I know that I have a heavenly home. The Psalmist crafted these words which express my thoughts. ...*I am always with you; you hold me by my right hand. You guide me with your counsel, and afterward you will take me into glory. Whom have I in heaven but you? And earth has nothing I desire besides you. My flesh and my heart may fail, but God is the strength of my heart and my portion forever.* **(Psalm 73:23-26)**

May you experience God's peace and enjoy eternity in His presence.

Shalom!

Acknowledgements

Thanks, and praise be to Father God, Jehovah Rophe, the Lord our healer, to Jesus Christ the Son, who took up our infirmities and carried our diseases and to the Holy Spirit who gives life to our mortal bodies.

...thanks be to God! He gives us the victory through our Lord Jesus Christ. (1 Corinthians 15:57)

Thanks also, to my dear wife, Desiree, and my family who stood by me in my darkest hours; to our local church, Living Waters, and to believers all over the world who prayed me through my ordeal.

My gratitude too, goes to my physicians: Dr Debbie Haasbroek, Dr Nick Michau, Dr Lance Coetzee, Dr Louis Hartley, Dr Sarita Retief, Dr Andrew McDonald, Dr Murray Augustyn, Dr Elizabeth Friend and Dr Carro de Witt. Thank you for your knowledge, experience and dedication. Without your help I wouldn't have made it.

Finally, a special word of thanks to Barbara Steenkamp who did the first and most needful and transformative editing which was followed by the efforts of the team at Kharis Publishing. My thanks to James Clement and the rest of the gang.

Appendix 1: Useful Resources

American Cancer Society https://www.cancer.org/

American Society of Clinical Oncology ® Cancer.Net, Doctor-Approved Patient Information https://www.cancer.net/

CANSA – The Cancer Association of South Africa https://cansa.org.za/

Drugs.com Know more. Be sure. https://www.drugs.com/

Livestrong.com https://www.livestrong.com/

Mayo Clinic https://www.mayoclinic.org/

MedicineNet https://www.medicinenet.com

Multiple Myeloma Research Foundation https://themmrf.org/

Myeloma Crowd Crowd Care Foundation https://www.myelomacrowd.org/

National Cancer Institute https://www.cancer.gov/

National Library of Medicine https://pubmed.ncbi.nlm.nih.gov/22301865/

Skin Cancer Foundation https://www.skincancer.org/

The National Center for Biotechnology Information https://www.ncbi.nlm.nih.gov/

Appendix 2: Daily Turmeric Shot

Take a shot of Turmeric daily after breakfast to mitigate against mucositis and inflammation of the colon.

- Pour 10 ml of honey (a tablespoon) into a small glass tumbler.

- Sprinkle ground cinnamon to cover the surface of the honey.

- Sprinkle some finely ground black pepper on the cinnamon (about half the quantity of the cinnamon).

- Add 5 ml of lemon juice (a teaspoon).

- Add 5g of ground turmeric (a heaped teaspoon) and stir mixture into a paste.

- Add a small amount of hot water to make mix liquid.

- Drink down in one or two gulps.

- Rinse mouth with a glass of water to prevent staining of teeth.

Notes:

If you are severely immune-suppressed use irradiated products. Black pepper increases the potency of turmeric; these two ingredients act synergistically. The mixture is more pleasant when drunk warm.

Appendix 3: Rooibos (Redbush) and Ginger Tea

Rooibos (Redbush) Tea is grown and produced in the Cedarberg region of the Western Cape Province of South Africa. It does not contain caffeine and has known healing properties.

The other ingredients: ginger and honey, also have known healing properties.

- Pour boiling water into a mug with a tea bag of Rooibos and a slice of fresh or frozen ginger.

- Simmer in a microwave at half power for about a minute. (This will help the tea and ginger to draw and become stronger).

- Add honey to sweeten to taste.

- Add a small amount of cold water to bring to a drinkable temperature.

- Drink and enjoy.

ABOUT THE AUTHOR

Pastor Phil, as he is affectionately known, has pastored Living Waters Church in Sabie, South Africa, for the past thirty-four years.

Recently retired from pastoral ministry, he is now pursuing a career as a Christian writer. As a person who has thrice survived cancer, he feels called to encourage and coach others fighting the disease.

Philip and Desirée have been happily married for 41 years. They have three children and three grandchildren.

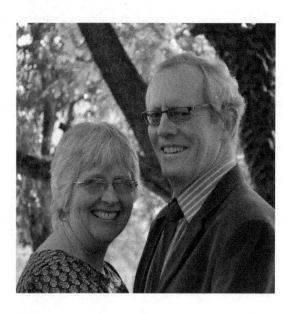

ABOUT
KHARIS PUBLISHING

KHARIS PUBLISHING is an independent, traditional publishing house with a core mission to publish impactful books, and channel proceeds into establishing mini-libraries or resource centers for orphanages in developing countries, so these kids will learn to read, dream, and grow. Every time you purchase a book from Kharis Publishing or partner as an author, you are helping give these kids an amazing opportunity to read, dream, and grow. Kharis Publishing is an imprint of Kharis Media LLC. Learn more at https://www.kharispublishing.com.

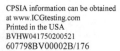

9 781637 460313